LOWER YOUR BLOOD PRESSURE

THE NO NONSENSE LIBRARY

NO NONSENSE HEALTH GUIDES

Women's Health and Fitness
A Diet for Lifetime Health
A Guide to Exercise and Fitness Equipment
How to Tone and Trim Your Trouble Spots
Stretch for Health
Unstress Your Life
Calories, Carbohydrates and Sodium
Permanent Weight Loss
All about Vitamins and Minerals
Your Emotional Health and Well-Being
Reducing Cholesterol
Soothe Your Aches and Pains
The Fiber Primer
Walk for Health

NO NONSENSE FINANCIAL GUIDES

NO NONSENSE REAL ESTATE GUIDES

NO NONSENSE LEGAL GUIDES

NO NONSENSE CAREER GUIDES

NO NONSENSE SUCCESS GUIDES

NO NONSENSE COOKING GUIDES

NO NONSENSE WINE GUIDES

NO NONSENSE PARENTING GUIDES

NO NONSENSE STUDENT GUIDES

NO NONSENSE AUTOMOTIVE GUIDES

NO NONSENSE PHOTOGRAPHY GUIDES

NO NONSENSE GARDENING GUIDES

NO NONSENSE HEALTH GUIDE®

LOWER YOUR BLOOD PRESSURE

Controlling Your Blood Pressure without Drugs

By the Editors of *PREVENTION* Magazine

Longmeadow Press

Notice

This book is intended as a reference volume only, not as a medical manual or guide to self-treatment. It is not intended as a substitute for the medical advice of physicians. The reader should regularly consult a physician in general, and particularly for any symptoms. If you suspect that you have a medical problem, we urge you to seek competent medical help. Keep in mind that exercise and nutritional needs vary from person to person, depending on age, sex, health status, and individual variations. The information here is intended to help you make informed decisions about your health, not as a substitute for any treatment that may have been prescribed by your doctor.

Lower Your Blood Pressure

Copyright © 1991 by Rodale Press, Inc. All rights reserved.
Cover Art © 1991 by Rodale Press, Inc. All rights reserved.

Published February 1991 by Longmeadow Press, 201 High Ridge Road, Stamford, CT 06904. No part of this book may be reproduced or used in any form or by any means, electronic or mechanical, including photocopying, recording, or any other information storage and retrieval system, without permission in writing from the publisher.

No Nonsense Health Guide is a trademark controlled by Longmeadow Press.

Library of Congress Cataloging-in-Publication Data

Lower your blood pressure : controlling your blood pressure without drugs
  / by the editors of Prevention magazine.
          p.   cm. — (No nonsense health guide)
      ISBN 0–681–41022–1 paperback
      1. Hypertension—Popular works.   2. Hypertension—Diet therapy.
3. Hypertension—Exercise therapy.   4. Hypertension—Psychosomatic
aspects.   I. Prevention (Emmaus, Pa.)   II. Series: No-nonsense health
guide.
   BC685.H8L69 1991
   616. 1'3206—dc20   90–25656
                                                                  CIP

Compiled and edited by Marcia Holman

Book design by Rodale Design Staff

Photographs by John P. Hamel, p. 54; Rodale Stock Images, pp. 5, 13, 25, 35, 49; Sally Shenk Ullman, pp. 26, 61, 73, 79.

Printed in the United States of America on acid-free paper ∞

0 9 8 7 6 5 4 3 2   paperback

Contents

New-Fashioned Blood Pressure Control

High blood pressure. This condition works a lot like a New York City mugger: It sneaks up on you. You go along minding your own business and then . . . BAM . . . your doctor tells you that you have hypertension.

Fifty million Americans are stalked by this silent killer. So if you have high blood pressure, you're not alone. If you are one of the victims, it simply means your blood pressure is in high throttle all the time. In other words, your blood courses through your veins and arteries with higher-than-average force. And with every little rise in blood pressure, you come closer to seriously endangering your health. With increased blood pressure, the arteries become less elastic, harder, thicker, and more susceptible to blockage. Thick, clogged arteries mean reduced blood flow to the vital organs, like your heart, brain, or kidneys. With too little blood flow to the heart, for example, you may have a heart attack. Too little blood to the brain and you may have a stroke. But the damage caused by hypertension occurs gradually, with no severe pain or other advance warning. Then, suddenly, the damage becomes all too apparent.

What's just as mysterious is why hypertension is twice as likely to strike blacks, or why it runs in families. Perhaps certain people release hormones that make their blood vessels clamp down more vigorously. Others may have kidneys that are unable to flush enough sodium from the body, and the more sodium you have in your system, the more fluid the body retains. This contributes to blood volume, raising blood pressure.

Although scientists are still uncertain why some people develop high blood pressure problems and others don't, they *are* sure about one thing: This puzzling disorder is the most treatable—and perhaps one of the most preventable—of all chronic ailments. Impressive evidence now indicates that while you may inherit a *tendency* to develop hypertension, you can take steps to avoid it. What's more, if you already have high blood pressure, taking costly or bothersome drugs may not be your only option. In fact, state-of-the-art blood pressure control involves dietary and lifestyle changes, not medicine alone.

Apparently, what you eat, whether or not you exercise, and how you deal with stress can influence blood pressure levels. Several studies have shown that a sizable number of people with mild hypertension can lower their blood pressure by reducing the fat and sodium in their diet, shedding excess weight, exercising regularly, and managing stress. What's more, other studies show that by making these lifestyle changes, people who've taken blood pressure medication for years can be weaned off drugs, or at least reduce their dosage.

Lower Your Blood Pressure is aimed at helping you make gradual changes in your daily habits that will protect your heart, strengthen your arteries, and get your blood flowing more freely. And the best part is, you don't have to turn your life upside down to get your blood pressure down. You'll learn easy ways to modify your diet so you can lose weight and cut fat and sodium. And you'll find tips for phasing in exercise, plus strategies for handling daily stress. Making these minor changes will be painless, but the effort will pay off quickly. In just a few weeks' time, you could ease your blood pressure down to a safe level and keep it there for the rest of your life.

Checking Your Blood Pressure: A Guide to What the Numbers Mean

High blood pressure can be like a time bomb ticking soundlessly within your body. Day after day, month after month, high-throttled blood pressure continues to overtax the arteries, severely battering them and harming the organs these blood vessels serve. High blood pressure speeds up atherosclerosis (hardening of the arteries), damages your nervous system, and overworks your heart.

This harm occurs without pain or warning symptoms, until one day, the damage becomes strikingly noticeable. If your high blood pressure is untreated and you are over 45, you are three times more likely to have a heart attack and seven times more likely to experience a stroke than those with normal blood pressure.

Fortunately, the high blood pressure "time bomb" within you can easily be defused, once it's detected. And the only sure way to detect it is to have your blood pressure taken. So don't wait another minute. Have your blood pressure taken today. It may just save your life.

Measuring your blood pressure is a simple procedure. Usually,

1

a doctor or nurse straps a rubber cuff around your upper arm, inflates it, and listens to your pulse through a stethoscope pressed against your artery at the elbow. As the cuff deflates, the blood moves through your arteries and a mercury-containing gauge registers the pressure.

Your blood pressure reading consists of two numbers—a higher number over a lower number. The higher number refers to systolic pressure, which is the maximum pressure put on the arteries when the heart is pumping. The lower number, the diastolic pressure, represents the minimum pressure, when the heart is resting between beats. Together, these numbers indicate the force exerted as your blood moves through your system.

A *normal* blood pressure reading is somewhere around 120 over 80. If your reading registers *more* than 140 over 90, you are considered to have mild hypertension, the medical term for slightly elevated blood pressure. Very high blood pressure, or severe hypertension, is 160 over 100 or more.

A Treatable Problem

If your readings fall above the normal range, don't panic. It doesn't mean you are stuck with hypertension for life. High blood pressure is the most treatable—and perhaps one of the most preventable—of all chronic ailments.

"Thirty years ago, relatively few people with hypertension could control their blood pressure," says Aram V. Chobanian, M.D., a member of the Joint National Committee on the Detection, Evaluation and Treatment of High Blood Pressure and director of the Cardiovascular Institute at Boston University Medical Center. "But now practically everyone can achieve some degree of control, and most can bring their pressure down to the normal range."

About 70 percent of all patients have mild hypertension—that is, their diastolic pressure (the bottom or lower reading) falls somewhere between 90 and 105. Don't be misled by the word *mild*. If your readings fall within the mild range, it's recommended that you consult your doctor and begin making dietary and lifestyle changes to get your blood pressure back to normal.

Even people with blood pressure readings *below* the 140/90 threshold may have reason to be concerned and should take action to lower their blood pressure.

"Research shows that there's a progressive increase in cardiovascular risk as systolic pressure rises above 130 and diastolic pressure goes above 85," says Dr. Chobanian. "People with diastolic pressure as low as 85 to 89 (the 'high normal' category) should act to bring their pressure under control, especially since a significant percentage of high normals eventually become severe hypertensives."

If your initial pressure is *very* high—160 over 100 or more—your doctor may prescribe a mild medication such as a diuretic. But even if you have been advised to take medication, making gradual lifestyle changes may help you reduce your dosage—and perhaps get your blood pressure under control so that eventually you won't have to take a single pill.

Once Is Not Enough

Do not start any treatment plan for high blood pressure until you have had several measurements taken. Hypertension cannot be accurately measured on the basis of a single reading. Put another way, *one* elevated blood pressure reading does not necessarily mean you have hypertension. A random sample of nearly 3,000 people, for example, found that hypertension was overestimated by as much as 30 percent when diagnosis was based on just one reading, compared with diagnosis after three separate readings.

Many factors can cause a false high reading. In fact, certain everyday events can make your blood pressure jump as much as 30 points during the day. Your heart may start thumping faster and your blood pressure building if you've just had a few cups of coffee or a run-in with your boss or made a mad dash to catch the bus. For some people, just the sight of the doctor's white coat can elevate their blood pressure. Research shows that, apparently, the anxiety some people feel at a doctor's office may account for their blood pressure reading that day. So have your blood pressure taken several times at the doctor's office and in another setting (say, at work on an uneventful day).

How High Is High?

You have hypertension if your top reading is above 140 or your bottom reading is above 90. However, you should start to take steps to lower your blood pressure even if you are in the high-normal range (that is, you have a systolic reading above 130 or a diastolic reading above 85).

Blood Pressure Reading	Classification
Systolic **(the top and higher reading)**	
Less than 140	Normal
140 to 159	Borderline isolated systolic hypertension
160 or higher	Isolated systolic hypertension
Diastolic **(the bottom and lower reading)**	
Less than 85	Normal
85 to 89	High normal
90 to 104	Mild hypertension
105 to 114	Moderate hypertension
115 or higher	Severe hypertension

The Pluses of Taking Your Own Blood Pressure

One of the best ways to get an accurate reading is to use a do-it-yourself home blood pressure kit. Taking your blood pressure in the relaxed privacy of your own home and at various times throughout the day helps you detect a consistently elevated blood pressure and can also *enhance* active participation in its treatment. If you have high blood pressure, you'll be encouraged by evidence that it's being controlled, and you'll be more likely to stay on your treatment program, according to the American Heart Association.

Home tests can help your doctor help you, too. Keeping careful records of home readings (including time, date, your body position, and what activities you're doing) helps your doctor to prescribe, evaluate, and adjust your treatment program. This is especially important for people trying drugless therapy, say doctors affiliated with the National High Blood Pressure Education Program and the National Institutes of Health, in Bethesda, Maryland.

Once you start monitoring your blood pressure on a regular basis, you may be surprised to discover that the numbers actually start to go down without making any other lifestyle changes! In fact, studies indicate that regular monitoring of blood pressure may be the easiest way to lower blood pressure.

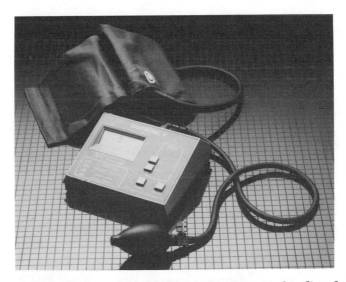

A home blood pressure kit is a smart investment. Studies show that for some people, monitoring their blood pressure regularly may be the only treatment needed. Apparently, just knowing you are going to take your blood pressure helps you relax; and it may be that the more you relax, the more you may ease down blood pressure.

When 40 people with mild cases of hypertension were sub-
jected to monitoring at 9-week intervals, their blood pressures were
lower after 18 weeks than those of a group of similar hypertensives
who attended classes either in muscle relaxation alone or in combination with biofeedback, exercise, and dietary changes.

Measuring may work its apparent magic in several ways. It
may serve as its own form of biofeedback as patients observe their
blood pressure on a regular basis. Or a placebo effect may exist:
As patients begin to expect monitoring to lower pressure, it does.
There's also the possibility that patients become more relaxed during the actual measurement process.

Go Lean and Lighten Your Blood Pressure

If you have a gradually expanding "spare tire" around your waistline, you may be jacking up your blood pressure.

Medical studies show that when body weight goes up, blood pressure goes up. On the average, a man's blood pressure jumps 6.5 points systolic for every 10 pounds of weight gain. A woman's pressure increases about half this amount.

"Our data suggest that overweight is one of the most powerful contributors to hypertension," says William B. Kannel, M.D., chief of preventive medicine and epidemiology at Boston University Medical Center. "We estimate that as many as 70 percent of the new cases of hypertension in young adults could be directly attributed to weight gain."

There are many theories to explain why, when you pile on the pounds, your blood pressure rises. One explanation may be that your sympathetic nervous system secretes increased adrenaline hormones as your weight goes up, resulting in elevated blood pressure. Another theory points the finger at additional fat cells, which decrease the effectiveness of insulin, a hormone that makes the body retain sodium. To compensate for the added cells, your body produces more insulin, resulting in increased sodium retention. And the more sodium retained in your body, the higher your blood pressure.

Some experts believe that excess pounds overload your heart—it has to work harder to pump enough blood to nourish your over-sized body. The more blood in your system, the more pressure it takes to circulate it through your arteries.

Drop Pounds and Drop Points

Even a weight gain of 10 pounds can boost your blood pressure several points.

If you drop the excess weight, on the other hand, you ease up on your heart . . . and your blood pressure. Losing weight is sometimes the only thing people need to do to drop their blood pressure to normal, experts say. "Weight loss is the single most important step to controlling blood pressure," according to Marvin Moser, M.D., clinical professor of medicine, Yale University School of Medicine, and author of *How to Control High Blood Pressure without Drugs.*

And the best news is that you don't necessarily have to lose it all! Researchers have found that weight loss can dramatically lower blood pressure *even if ideal weight isn't reached.* One estimate is that obese people can decrease their blood pressure an average of 8 to 10 points (systolic or diastolic) by losing 20 to 25 pounds.

For every 2 pounds you lose, studies show, you can lower both your systolic and diastolic blood pressure by one point. Lose enough weight, and you could drop enough points to take you right out of the hypertension category.

Although studies indicate that weight loss through diet or exercise alone can reduce blood pressure, most experts agree that the healthiest strategy is a program combining both diet and exercise.

Slim Down Your Meals

The simplest way to get rid of excess weight is to trim the extra calories from your daily meals. Fortunately, you can whittle off the excess pounds without going on a rigid diet. "You don't have to eat bowls of boiled rice to get your blood pressure down," says Robert Rowan, M.D., of New York Medical School. In fact, a gradual, commonsense change is more likely to lead to permanent weight loss. A diet that causes you to lose one to two pounds a week allows your body to adjust to the new, lower level of calories.

Begin a food diary. Keeping track of all your meals (including your snacks) will help you spot high-calorie foods you consume almost without thinking. Your diary may reveal the corn chips you munch while watching TV, the syrup you put on your pancakes, the butter on your potato, the high-calorie dressing on your salad. When you see what you actually eat each day, you can start to replace the calorie-laden foods with lighter fare.

You can, for example, snack on air-popped popcorn, a low-calorie alternative to chips. Or sweeten your pancakes with "lite" syrup or apple butter, both of which have fewer calories than regular syrup and butter. You may enjoy dressing your salad with low-fat cottage cheese that's been whipped in a blender instead of Thousand Island dressing. Your goal is to ease out the sugar and trim the fat from your diet.

Limit the bad fats. Even if you're not overweight, reducing fat intake can help you reduce your blood pressure.

If you eat too much fat—especially saturated fat, the kind found in dairy products and red meats—the cholesterol level in your blood can soar, elevating your blood pressure. Evidently, surplus cholesterol seeps into cracks in arteries worn thin from the buffeting force of blood coursing through them. Waxy clumps of plaque form, the blood vessels narrow, and your blood pressure rises.

One notable study—one of a long line of similar investigations—suggests that it may actually be possible for people to lower their blood pressure by cutting back on (or changing the type of) fat in their diet. In the three-month trial, middle-aged men with normal blood pressure followed either a low-fat diet (25 percent of calories from fat, with equal amounts of polyunsaturated and saturated fats) or a more typically American diet (about 40 percent of calories from fat, mostly saturated). They all consumed the same kinds of foods, but the low-fat group ate leaner fare—like meat trimmed of fat, low-fat milk, and margarine. And in line with the results of other studies, there was a 9 percent drop in blood pressure in the group that was on the low-fat diet.

Researcher James M. Iacono, Ph.D., director of the U.S. Department of Agriculture's Western Human Nutrition Research Center in San Francisco, says that the data he gathered suggest a cause for the decrease in blood pressure. "The bodies of the men in the low-fat group excreted (got rid of) 4 percent more sodium and 11 percent more potassium than those in the normal-fat group," he says. "The excretion of these two minerals, one of which, sodium, is known to sometimes raise blood pressure with higher daily intake, may be what triggers the reductions in the blood pressure."

If such low-fat diets can pull down blood pressure as well as research suggests, they may soon become as crucial as low-salt eating in the nondrug treatment of hypertension. "Until scientists can define the most effective low-fat diet for reducing blood pressure," says Dr. Iacono, "the wisest approach is to follow the current recommendations to reduce overall fat to about 30 percent of total calories and maintain equal amounts of polyunsaturated and saturated fats."

Switch to the good fats.   Not all fats are bad for your blood pressure. Research indicates that polyunsaturated and monounsaturated fats, which are usually found in fish, vegetable oils, seeds, and nuts, may help lower blood pressure and, in effect, neutralize the negative effects of saturated fats, which usually turn up in protein-rich foods of animal origin, such as red meat, eggs, and full-fat dairy products.

In a pilot study of healthy people in Italy, Finland, and the United States, researchers discovered that the level of dietary linoleic acid—a polyunsaturated fat—was associated with incidence of high blood pressure. There were more hypertensives among the Finnish population than among the Italians and Americans. The Finns consumed more saturated and less polyunsaturated fats.

Fat Substitutions at Your Fingertips

Go for the Good Fats (Substitute for bad fats when possible; eat in moderation.)	Avoid the Bad Fats (Don't exceed 8 servings per week.)
Dairy Low-fat cheeses (cottage cheese, part-skim mozzarella, ricotta); low-fat yogurt; 1%, 2%, or skim milk (or, if you're not quite ready for skim milk, try cutting whole milk with 25% skim—later raise to 50%), tofu ice cream	High-fat cheeses (Brie, cheddar, Neufchâtel, Swiss, etc.); whole-fat yogurt; whole-fat milk, cream; ice cream
Meat and Protein Poultry, skinned and visible fat removed; fish; shellfish; dried beans and peas; egg substitutes and egg whites; tofu and tempeh	Red meat, all visible fat trimmed before cooking; organ meats; egg yolks; processed meats
Salad Oils and Cooking Fat Corn, cottonseed, safflower, soybean, sunflower oils	Bacon fat; lard; shortening; hydrogenated vegetable oil
Spreads Margarine, peanut butter without hydrogenated fat	Butter; "regular" peanut butter

When a group of Finns aged 40 to 50 were placed on a low-fat diet high in polyunsaturated fats and low in saturated fats, blood pressures dropped significantly, even when salt consumption wasn't reduced. When they returned to their old eating habits, their old blood pressures returned, too.

What's the story? Dr. Ianoco and other researchers have one theory. They believe polyunsaturated fats lower blood pressure because when they're metabolized by the body, they yield a substance that is essential for making prostaglandins. These are fatty acids that seem to control pressure by aiding in the sloughing off of water and salt from the kidneys.

Another friendly fat is eicosapentanoic acid, one of the omega-3 fatty acids, found in mackerel and other marine fish.

West German researchers have found that including mackerel in the diet lowered blood pressure among men with mild hypertension. Their pressure reverted to its original high level only when the men went back to their old diets, which were low in fish and high in cold cuts.

Follow a Fat-Free Formula with Pleasure

There are really only two important things to remember when you're changing the fat content of your diet to try to lower your blood pressure.

First, keep your total fat intake to less than 30 percent of your total calories. Second, get more than half of your fat as polyunsaturates, monounsaturates, and omega-3 fatty acids—the fats found in most vegetable oils like safflower and olive oils, and in some varieties of fish.

It's easier to follow this formula than you may think. You don't have to struggle to give up your favorite foods. Think about reducing fats and substituting low-fat alternatives rather than eliminating fat entirely.

Here are some ideas that help you trim the fat and still savor the rich taste and texture of the foods you love.

- Choose low-fat dairy products. Select low-fat and nonfat milk over whole milk; low-fat yogurt and evaporated skim milk instead of heavy cream. Substitute part-skim ricotta, part-skim mozzarella, and low-fat cottage cheese for high-fat cheddar or cream cheese.
- Meet Amazing Mayo. This creamy-smooth slim mayo is delicious and easy to prepare. Puree ½ cup (4 ounces) soft tofu, 1 teaspoon white vinegar, 1 teaspoon lemon

juice, ¼ teaspoon dry mustard, and a pinch of cayenne pepper in a blender or food processor.

- Trade sour cream for yogurt to top your baked potato, to replace the mayo in tuna salad, and to substitute for cream toppings. If you're sweet on sour cream, here's how to give up the fat and keep the flavor. Puree ¼ cup buttermilk, ½ cup nonfat cottage cheese, and 2 teaspoons lemon juice in a blender until smooth. Transfer to a medium bowl and stir in snipped chives or other minced fresh herbs. You can serve it as a dip or as a topping for steamed vegetables.
- Dress for success. Make a thick and creamy fat-free salad dressing by whisking ½ teaspoon freshly squeezed lemon juice into ½ cup nonfat yogurt. Stir

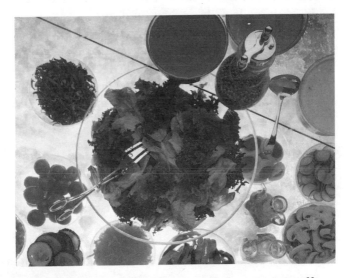

Eating salads helps you slim down and shave points off your blood pressure, but only if you skip the high-fat cold cuts, creamy dressings, and salty relishes that show up as extras. Pile on lean-and-mean veggies, low-cal cottage cheese, crunchy seeds, and sprouts. Drizzle lightly with olive oil, a lighter, "good fat" that can lower blood pressure.

in dill and chopped cucumber to taste. For a Thousand Island-type dressing, fold 2 tablespoons tomato paste into the above dressing. Add minced garlic, pickles, shallots, and celery to taste.

- Lighten up cream sauces and soups with evaporated milk instead of heavy cream. Or use warm mashed potatoes as a fat-free thickener. If you're making a sauce, just heat the milk and whisk in enough potatoes to get the desired consistency.
- Microwave onions and garlic before adding them to your recipe. You'll soften them and bring out their full flavor without using a bit of fat.
- For dessert, try fruit ices or delicious sorbets instead of ice cream.
- Trim the fat off red meats, and take the skin off poultry. When possible, substitute poultry for red meat. Try chili made with chicken, and meat loaf made with ground turkey.
- Make magic marinades. Here is one fat-free recipe for chicken: Combine the juice and pulp of 1 lemon with 1 clove garlic (minced) and 1 teaspoon dried oregano. Add 1 pound skinless, boneless chicken breasts and marinate for at least an hour. Grill as usual or sauté in a nonstick frying pan.
- Slim your stuffing. Never cook stuffing in the bird. That way, it won't absorb any fat that drips from the poultry. Get that great oven-roasted flavor by moistening the stuffing ingredients with fat-free chicken or turkey stock.
- Alternate your meat meals with fish—especially the darker, ocean fish such as mackerel, tuna, salmon, and sardines.
- Eat lean vegetarian dishes when you can. Try meatless lasagna or pasta with low-fat sauce as an entrée. Choose red sauces versus white, creamy sauces.
- Banish butter. Switch to margarine made with corn or soybean oil. Better yet, choose one of the light, whipped tub brands. The softer the margarine, the less hydro-

genation it has undergone. Hydrogenation is a chemical process that makes fat saturated, and saturated fat is exactly what you want to avoid.

- Spread fruit butters. They're smooth and silky with absolutely no fat. Try spiced apple butter on a bran muffin or peach butter on oat-bran toast.
- Avoid snacks, cereals, and all prepared foods that list hydrogenated oils or nonspecific vegetable oil as an ingredient. Unspecified oil could turn out to be coconut or palm—two oils that are high in saturated fat.
- Switch to low-fat snacks like pretzels, fruit, or carrot sticks.

Watch Your Blood Pressure Go Down, Down

Once you've gotten into the habit of eating low-fat meals and exercising regularly, you will see that spare tire around your middle start to deflate a little and your blood pressure start to go down.

Go back and have your blood pressure checked. If your levels have dropped, congratulate yourself. But now's not the time to slack off. You need to stick to your low-blood-pressure regime to keep your blood pressure low and within the normal range.

C H A P T E R
T H R E E

A Consumer's Guide to Foods That Battle High Blood Pressure

Our primitive ancestors didn't know about gourmet cooking, taco stands, or cookies shaped like animals. They never tasted a cream-filled éclair drenched in Dutch chocolate. Savory french fries never touched their lips.

Today, we enjoy a bounty of rich, quick, and tasty foods. Yet we pay for these recent acquisitions with our health. And the price is often high blood pressure.

Part of the reason so many people have high blood pressure is that our diets have become out of tune with our body chemistry, say experts such as Louis Tobian, M.D., head of hypertension programs at the University of Minnesota in Minneapolis.

Back when people lived in caves, a typical meal (they were lucky to *have* a meal) consisted of fruits, vegetables, and nuts. These meals were brimming with fiber and nutrients but contained scant amounts of salt and fat. Since we need a small amount of salt (sodium, to be more accurate) and fat to maintain health and life, our bodies learned how to conserve sodium and store fat.

At the same time, while our bodies were learning how to conserve fat and sodium, they did not learn how to store potassium. And potassium helps counteract the harmful effects of excess sodium.

Today, the typical American diet is nearly the exact opposite of our earlier meals. In place of the vegetables, fruits, and other fiber-rich, nutrient-dense staples, we feast on savory steaks, creamy milkshakes, salads drenched in oily dressings, crunchy nacho chips—all foods loaded with salt and fat, and often lacking in adequate vitamins and minerals.

And while our nutritional environment changed radically, our body chemistry didn't. Suddenly we were eating a lot of fat, which our bodies—programmed to suspect a famine around every corner—gratefully stored. Suddenly we were eating a lot of salt, and our bodies salted it away. Suddenly we were eating less potassium.

One result of this modern diet is that rising numbers of Americans have become plagued with a host of modern conditions—and high blood pressure is among the most common, affecting 50 million Americans. Excess sodium constricts the blood vessels, while an overabundance of fat can clog the arteries. And constricted blood vessels and blocked arteries can boost the blood pressure to dangerous levels.

Wage Dietary War on High Blood Pressure

Fortunately, we have the know-how to fight high blood pressure. How? Not through the miracles of modern chemistry, but by choosing the best wholesome foods Mother Nature has to offer. Unlike the dinosaurs that died out millions of years ago, we can create a diet that helps us cooperate with our bodies instead of fighting them. We can learn to skip the additives, like salt and buttery oils and fats, and put back the minerals and nutrients that modern food processing has taken away.

And more and more doctors are suggesting dietary changes as the first, and sometimes the only, front-line treatment for high blood pressure.

"Research shows that modifying your eating habits really can work," says Cleaves Bennett, M.D., medical director of the Los

Angeles InnerHealth Clinic and co-author of *The Control Your High Blood Pressure Cookbook*. "Dietary changes help some people avoid ever having to take blood pressure drugs, and they help others decrease their dosage," Dr. Bennett says.

Researchers with the Hypertension Control Program (HCP) in Chicago and Minneapolis studied a group of men and women aged 35 and older with mildly elevated blood pressure. Some of the subjects stopped their medications and began a diet to lose weight and restrict their use of sodium and alcohol. Others discontinued their drugs without changing their food habits in any way. After four years, 39 percent of the first group had stayed off their medication and were still in the normal blood pressure range compared with only 5 percent of the second group.

Lowering blood pressure without drugs eliminates the drugs' immediate side effects and long-term health risks, say the researchers. They also point out that you have a better chance of lowering blood pressure by nutritional means, without medication, if you have less-severe hypertension to begin with. It also helps if you're not too overweight or consuming extremely high levels of sodium or alcohol when you start the treatment.

Don't expect instant results once you change your diet. "Modifying your eating habits needs to be given a chance—two months minimum and up to a year for people with severe high blood pressure," says Dr. Bennett. "Both patient and doctor need to be committed to making the changes work." (And, of course, any changes, especially reductions in medication, should have medical supervision.)

Just what foods compose a diet for a healthier future? Here are the experts' recommendations, along with the latest research findings on nutrients that really work against high blood pressure.

Get Thee to the Garden

Succulent vegetables with fresh-from-the-garden taste—leafy green lettuce, potatoes bursting with flavor. Juicy, sun-ripened fruits—sweet bananas, mouth-watering melons, chewy apricots. Tantalizing whole-grain breads. Crunchy nuts. Savory beans. Experts say that the cornucopia of vegetables, fruits, and grains are the foot soldiers in your battle against high blood pressure.

In fact, we may be better off making vegetables the center-piece of our meals. Studies have shown that vegetarians have lower blood pressure than the general population—10 to 15 points lower for both systolic and diastolic pressures.

But it's not the absence of meat in their diet that protects vegetarians from high blood pressure, says Frank M. Sacks, M.D., of Harvard Medical School. He suspects that it's the higher levels of minerals—magnesium, calcium, and potassium—in the fruits and vegetables vegetarians eat that protect them from high blood pressure.

These minerals form a mighty trio when it comes to fighting high blood pressure. Each in some way helps regulate the function of the blood vessels and maintain a proper balance of sodium in the body. Fortunately, magnesium, calcium, and potassium are often found together in foods. So if you select foods loaded in one mineral, chances are you'll be getting a healthy helping of the other minerals as well.

Let's take a closer look at how these prime blood pressure minerals work and how you can work them—as well as other important nutrients—into your daily diet.

Make the calcium connection.   Only recently have researchers noted that some cheese and milk lovers seem to have lower blood pressure. Now, they are pinpointing just who benefits from additional calcium.

"Additional calcium seems to work best for people who are hypertensive and salt-sensitive," says Lawrence Resnick, M.D., of the Cardiovascular Center at New York Hospital–Cornell Medical Center. These are people whose blood pressure goes up 5 percent or more when they switch from a low- to a high-salt diet. In one study, Dr. Resnick found that adding 2,000 milligrams a day of calcium to the high-salt diets of salt-sensitive people blunted salt's blood-pressure-raising effects. One-third to one-half of all people with high blood pressure, and especially blacks and older people, are salt-sensitive, Dr. Resnick says.

"The present study indicates that the more salt elevates blood pressure, the more calcium lowers it," Dr. Resnick says. So if salt is bad for you, calcium's good for you.

Low-fat dairy products are excellent choices for calcium. Other good calcium sources are sardines, salmon, leafy greens, and nuts.

Make much ado about magnesium.   What do buckwheat pancakes, almonds, and bananas have in common? They're all good sources of magnesium, a mineral that tempers both steel and blood vessels. "Magnesium is probably one of the most promising and least-used minerals when it comes to blood-pressure control," says Burton Altura, M.D., Ph.D., a leading blood pressure researcher.

One study, conducted by Honolulu Heart Program researchers, clearly shows magnesium's importance in blood pressure control. The scientists examined 61 different factors in the diets of healthy, older men. Magnesium came out on top, having the strongest link between high intake and low blood pressure.

How does magnesium work? The exact mechanism is unknown, but it is believed that magnesium helps your heart to beat smoothly and helps blood vessels remain open and relaxed, lowering your blood pressure. Furthermore, magnesium seems to help regulate the calcium supply in the cells of the vascular system. Magnesium and calcium work as partners, helping the blood vessels contract and relax.

How to meet your quota. Many mineral researchers think an average-size man should be getting about 420 to 475 milligrams of magnesium a day to make up for what he loses—and to help protect him from developing high blood pressure as he ages. That's about 125 to 150 milligrams a day more than most men get.

Avoid overprocessed food. In fact, most of us fall short of the recommended allowances of magnesium by 350 to 450 milligrams a day. One reason? Overprocessed food. Take, for example, the sandwich bread you select. If your sandwich is made with white bread, it's likely that most of the magnesium has been lost when the flour was refined and processed. You'd be better off selecting whole-grain bread for your sandwich. Bread made with whole wheat flour gives you five times as much magnesium as bread made with white flour.

Don't soften your water. If your plumbing is hooked up to a water softener, you may be extracting an important blood pressure mineral from your water along with the other minerals you don't want. Preserve the magnesium in your water supply—make sure you don't hook up your water softener to the water you use for drinking or cooking.

Boiling is a no-no. Boiling vegetables can leach out their magnesium: one-half to three-fourths of the magnesium content of carrots, celery, and parsnips can be found in their cooking water. Green vegetables generally contain adequate amounts of magnesium, but they should be steamed, baked, or broiled.

To sum it all up, a magnesium-rich meal would contain one or more of these foods: whole-grain bread, bananas, brown rice, spinach, corn, fresh fruit or green vegetables, molasses, or bran. White bread or cake, white rice, and boiled rice, on the other hand, are magnesium-poor.

Pass the potassium, please.   Potassium performs countless vital functions in the body. But in its missions, potassium is intimately and mysteriously linked to the activities of sodium. The two substances carry on a sort of unceasing tug-of-war across the walls of the cells. At stake is the delicate electrical and chemical balance of the body.

When sodium wins, the cells contain more water, and potassium is dumped into the urine for excretion. When potassium wins, the cells get rid of sodium and water. Though sodium plays its own role in the body's chemistry, you only need minute amounts—and anything above that can be considered a potassium burglar, robbing the system of a vital mineral and sending it on its way where it will do nobody any good.

Various studies of this cellular shoot-out have turned up intriguing new indications that potassium may somehow act as a shield against sodium-induced high blood pressure. In one study, a group of 16 people with mild hypertension and a group with normal blood pressure received two different diets, each for a period of 12 weeks. During the first 12 weeks, both groups ate their normal diet, plus sodium tablets. During the second period, their normal diets were supplemented with potassium, and they were instructed to avoid excessively salty foods and not to add salt while cooking or at the table.

The high-sodium diet produced a slow rise in blood pressure in both groups. But during the high-potassium/low-sodium diet, both systolic and diastolic blood pressure fell sharply and significantly in the hypertensive group in contrast to small rises in the nomotensive (healthy) group, according to the researchers.

A month after the study had ended and the people *had* resumed their regular eating habits, both groups were tested one final time. The hypertensives' blood pressure had shot right back up again. The researchers concluded that the key factor in the startling drop in pressure during the high-potassium/low-sodium diet had been the increased potassium, since the regular diets included only a marginal rise in sodium but a much greater decline in potassium.

Some researchers even suggest that potassium's gentle power may have an effect on nearly everybody, even those without high blood pressure.

Potassium does help counteract sodium's negative effects, says George D. Webb, Ph.D., a professor in the Department of Physics and Biophysics at the University of Vermont College of Medicine and co-author of *The K Factor: Reversing and Preventing High Blood Pressure Without Drugs*. (K is the chemical symbol for potassium.) "We believe there's a clear benefit when you get three times as much potassium as sodium," says Dr. Webb. "If you're on a low-salt diet and getting two grams of sodium (2 grams of sodium equals 5 grams of table salt) per day, then you should get 6 grams of potassium."

Stock up on K-factor foods. To meet the 3:1 potassium/sodium ratio, most people need to cut their sodium intake to 2,000 milligrams or less a day. And they must make a conscious effort to eat more potassium-rich foods like fresh fruit, fish, nuts, leafy greens, whole grains, and potatoes.

How do you know if you're getting enough potassium? "It's hard to avoid potassium if you eat plenty of natural foods," says Dr. Webb. Bananas, oranges, and potatoes are packed with potassium. One orange, for example, contains 263 milligrams of the mineral. A potato has 130 times more potassium than sodium—and it's one food you can work into breakfast, lunch, or dinner. Try a potato pancake tomorrow for breakfast. You can even make a baked potato your lunch or dinner entrée—pile it with steamed vegetables and melt some part-skim mozzarella on top.

Fresh food is best. When you buy canned or frozen fruits or vegetables, you may actually be reversing the sodium/potassium balance. For example, a cup of raw peas contains 458 milligrams of potassium and just 3 milligrams of sodium. Compare that to when those same peas are canned: salt added during the process raises the sodium level to 588 milligrams (a nearly 200-fold increase) and the potassium is roughly halved, down to 239 milligrams. That's to say nothing about what happens to the proportions when the peas hit the dinner table dressed in table salt and salted butter!

Monitor your medications. Some drugs force the body to excrete potassium. If you are taking blood pressure medicines, make sure you eat potassium-rich foods each meal.

Pick up a six-pack of vitamin C.   Soft drinks are loaded with sodium. But when you switch to orange juice you get two bonuses—not only a drink that's low in sodium and high in potassium but one that has a wallop of vitamin C. A group of Japanese researchers has suggested that high vitamin C intake may, in fact, help prevent high blood pressure from developing.

The researchers tested a group of healthy men (aged 30 to 39) to determine both their blood pressure and their blood levels of vitamin C. They found that the higher the vitamin C levels, the lower the incidence of high blood pressure. These results, say the researchers, could help explain why some populations with high dietary intake of vitamin C have a low mortality rate from heart disease and atherosclerosis, or hardening of the arteries.

In addition to citrus fruits, melons provide hefty amounts of vitamin C. Round, luscious casabas; juicy, sweet honeydews; tangy cantaloupes—all are loaded with vitamin C as well as potassium, a mineral that can get sweated away on sweltering days, or whenever you work up a sweat.

On sweltering days, try a cool melon cocktail. Take a cantaloupe, cut it in slices, and remove the skin. Now pare the slices into chunks and feed them one at a time into the blender. The result? Two cups of a refreshing, bright orange drink with a thick creamy head that's better still when chilled and served in frosted glasses.

Don't hold the onions.   Or the garlic. Studies show that these two pungent bulbs contain substances that may offer protection against that demon of modern, fast-paced life, high blood pressure.

According to Moses Attrep, Jr., Ph.D., formerly a chemist at East Texas State University, it may be a hormonelike substance he isolated in yellow onions called prostaglandin A-1, which also occurs in the human kidney. When injected into humans and animals, prostaglandin A-1 lowers blood pressure, at least for brief periods.

The Japanese and Chinese have used garlic to lower blood pressure for centuries. Its effect is possibly similar to that of onions, since it, too, may contain prostaglandins.

White-skinned garlic has the strongest flavor; pinkish or purplish garlic is milder.

The problem is, even mild garlic has an odor only another garlic eater could love. And, according to most researchers, garlic that's "deodorized" by heat treatment has no beneficial effects.

But here's some good news. At least one form of prepared garlic seems to retain its ability to lower blood fats. It's an odor-modified, cold-aged product from Japan, called Kyolic. And according to studies, it seems to work with half the odor.

Choose the Friendly Fats

Once you have made adjustments in your salt/potassium ratio in your meals, you should begin making adjustments in the kinds of fats you eat.

Butter, bacon fat, oils—all the fats we eat affect blood pressure because they are used by our bodies to make hormones known as prostaglandins. Some prostaglandins lower blood pressure, and

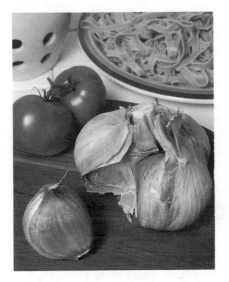

Garlic was once worn as a talisman to ward off evil spirits. Some experts now believe this pungent bulb could stave off hypertension. Garlic contains the same hormonelike substance found in yellow onions; when this substance was isolated from onions and injected into humans, blood pressure dropped to healthier levels.

whether the body manufactures these depends on which "building materials" it has on hand.

To change the fat content of your diet, keep your total fat intake to less than 30 percent of your total calories. That's most easily done by cutting back on saturated fats, the so-called bad fats—butter, margarine, oils, hard cheeses, fatty meats, and other concentrated fat sources.

Of the fat you do consume, make sure that more than half of it comes in the form of polyunsaturates, monounsaturates, and omega-3 fatty acids. All these fats appear to have blood-pressure-lowering effects. Among polyunsaturated oils, choose those high in linoleic acid—safflower and sunflower-seed oils. (Linoleic acid is used to produce the pressure-lowering prostaglandins.) Get monounsaturated fats from tasty olive and peanut oils. Omega-3 fatty acids, the oils found in such fish as salmon and mackerel and in shellfish and some vegetable oils (canola, for example), also seem to reduce blood pressure, at least when these fats are substituted for saturated fats.

Here are some ways to stock up on the "friendly fats":

Go Greek or Italian.   Translation: Make dishes using olive oil. If you've already switched to olive oil because you've heard of its cholesterol-busting prowess, you may be getting a healthy bonus. In one comprehensive study, olive oil was also linked to lower blood pressure and reduced blood-sugar levels.

The study took place in Italy, where residents run a low risk of coronary disease. Nearly 5,000 Italian men and women aged 20 to 59 were asked what kinds of fats and oils they used in their food and how frequently they used them. The study confirmed that those who used olive oil regularly had significantly lower cholesterol. It also found that their blood pressure was 2.5 percent lower (unlike those who used polyunsaturated fats, who showed no reduction in this heart-disease risk factor), and their blood sugar levels were 6.6 percent lower in men.

No one really knows how olive oil might do this, but Maurizio Trevisan, M.D., of the School of Medicine at State University of New York at Buffalo speculates, "Monounsaturated fats (like olive oil) may affect metabolism and production of insulin, which could explain the beneficial effect on both blood pressure and glucose levels."

So add olive oil to your daily menu whenever possible. Drizzle this "liquid gold" on salads. Use in all your pasta sauces. Saute your vegetables in a tablespoon of olive oil and fresh herbs. If you don't want to use olive oil straight, try mixing some with your regular vegetable oil.

But don't get carried away. Olive oil is, after all, pure fat. In excess, any fat can promote obesity, and obesity is associated with higher blood pressure levels.

Substitute a fish dish.   Mackerel and other marine fish like tuna, salmon, and shellfish contain eicosapentanoic acid, one of the omega-3 fatty acids. Researchers have shown that an easy-to-follow diet rich in this type of good fat can lower blood pressure in people with mild hypertension.

Researchers from the Central Institute for Cardiovascular Research in West Germany gave cans of mackerel with tomatoes to men who had mild hypertension and who didn't usually eat much fish. For two weeks, the men ate a daily diet that included two cans of the mackerel. Then they switched to eating just three cans of the fish per week, and followed that regimen for eight months. After that, they went back to their normal diet for two months.

After the first dietary period, the men's triglyceride levels, cholesterol levels, blood pressure, and blood-clotting tendency dropped significantly. And their levels of HDL-cholesterol (the kind thought to be beneficial) increased. During the second dietary period, when the amount of mackerel was cut back, all of these measurements returned to their initial levels, except blood pressure. That remained significantly lower and didn't return to the initial level until the men went back to their old habits—a diet low in fish and high in cold cuts and meat.

How about designating Monday, Wednesday, and Friday fish days at your house? Browse through your cookbook for tasty shell-fish dishes. Toss salmon chunks into your favorite cold pasta salad. Tuck a tuna pita sandwich in your lunchbox. And next time you're dining out, scan the menu for a mackerel dish.

Choose Fiber in All Its Forms

Perhaps you've started eating a high-fiber cereal as a hedge against heart attack. But did you know that your healthy habit may also be doing your blood pressure a favor?

In one study, when subjects ate three times the dietary fiber for a two-week period, their average blood pressure dropped ten percent. Researchers speculate that fiber helps your body produce less insulin. And insulin is the hormone that helps your body retain salt.

Another reason why fiber may help bring down high blood pressure is that it helps counteract an overabundance of saturated fats and reduce cholesterol. According to some researchers, fiber may escort the bad cholesterol out of your body before it can clog up your arteries. Less clogging cholesterol helps keep your arteries wide and open, allowing blood to flow more effortlessly. The more freely your blood flows, the lower your blood pressure.

It's fairly easy to work fiber into all your meals since Mother Nature packs a hefty dose of the stuff in practically all of her plant foods.

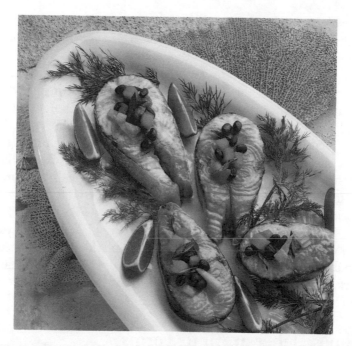

When you trade your beef steak for a salmon steak, you're trading a blood-pressure-boosting fat for a fat that lowers your blood pressure. Salmon, mackerel, and other marine fish are rich in omega-3 fatty acids, which have been shown to lower blood pressure just a few weeks after adding them to the diet.

You're probably already familiar with fiber in vegetables and fruits as well as grains such as whole wheat, oat bran, rice, and rye. But don't limit your grain intake to eating bread and cereal. Experiment. Toss wheat germ into soups, stews, or on top of salads. Dredge your poultry in an oat-bran seasoning. Mix rice bran into meat loaves or croquettes. Or try a refreshing cold rice, tomato, and vegetable salad to cool you off on sizzling summer days.

And give other grains a whirl. Buckwheat pancakes have a delicious old-fashioned nutty flavor. Bulgur, a familiar accompaniment to many Middle Eastern dishes, is amazingly versatile and can make a hearty addition to bread dough and other baked goods. Use it as an extender in meat or eat it plain.

Don't forget about beans—red, white, and navy beans, that is. They are excellent sources of fiber and can be included in dozens of recipes. Have a spicy bowl of chili for lunch. Or a crunchy, sprouted mung bean salad for supper.

25 All-Star Foods for Blood Pressure Control

With a little creativity, it's easy to include these blood-pressure-busting foods in your daily diet.

Feast on . . .	Blood-Pressure-Lowering Benefits
Fruits Bananas, apricots, oranges, raisins, and strawberries	Good sources of potassium and/or magnesium. Low in fat.
Vegetables Potatoes, spinach, sweet potatoes, Swiss chard, and tomatoes	Good sources of potassium and/or magnesium. Low in fat.
Fish Salmon, mackerel, tuna, and sardines	Good sources of polyunsaturated and omega-3 fats. Low in saturated fats.
Grains, Beans, Nuts Barley, brown rice, red kidney beans, tofu, almonds, and peanuts	Good sources of potassium and/or magnesium. Low in fat.
Oils Canola, olive, peanut, sunflower, and safflower oil	High in polyunsaturates or monounsaturates.

Sock It to Salt and Save Your Arteries

Salt. It does for food what bubbles do for champagne. It adds that extra zing that livens up everything from soup to nuts. Without salt, food can taste a little less tantalizing, a little more flat.

Even so, salt is one seasoning you should probably not invite to your next meal. The reason? Salt is an enemy to hypertensives and a suspicious character for people with normal blood pressure.

Sodium has been indicted as a prime suspect in high blood pressure on the basis of three kinds of circumstantial evidence. First, people who live in societies whose members eat very little salt rarely have high blood pressure, while people who live in societies where there is high salt intake (like the U.S.) frequently have high blood pressure. Second, animals with a genetic tendency toward high blood pressure ultimately develop this condition if they eat more salt than the body actually requires. This fact strongly implies that the same thing happens to people who, because their parents have hypertension, are predisposed to the disease.

Third, and even more convincing, studies have found that

people with high blood pressure have more sodium in the walls of their blood vessels than do people with normal blood pressure.

The salt/blood-pressure connection is more dangerous for some people than for others. A few people (the "salt resistant") can consume as much as 15 grams of salt a day (10 grams daily is the American average) without a significant jump in blood pressure. Others (the "salt sensitive") can get a rise in pressure with a much lower amount. And as far as we know, one-third to one-half of all adults may be in this sensitive group.

If you're salt sensitive, your kidneys may be unable to flush enough sodium from your body. And the more sodium you have in your system, the more fluid your body retains. The blood vessels become waterlogged and constrict; your blood pressure soars.

Are *You* Salt Sensitive?

Researchers have recently devised tests that can tell you whether you are salt sensitive, but the tests aren't widely available yet. Researchers do know, however, that if high blood pressure runs in your family, there's a good chance you're one of the susceptible people. They have also discovered that sensitivity to sodium increases as people get older.

"There's no way to know if you're salt sensitive other than putting yourself on a low-sodium diet and seeing what effect that has on your blood pressure," says Norman Kaplan, M.D., head of the hypertension section at the University of Texas Southwestern Medical School in Dallas.

If eating *more* sodium raises blood pressure, eating less should *lower* it. And to a great degree, cutting down on sodium does help enormously. One study reported that among 16 patients given only dietary advice—including the dictum to cut down on salt—12 lowered their blood pressure significantly after two months of cutting back their intake by 40 percent.

Some people taking blood pressure medication may even be able to temporarily discontinue their drugs by restricting sodium. Researchers studied 496 hypertensives who had successfully controlled their high blood pressure with drugs for some time. During the study, one group continued to take their medication while the other stopped; in place of medication they were put on a low-salt diet. They found that 77.8 percent of the people with mild hypertension who were not overweight successfully controlled their blood pressure for at least a year when they restricted sodium.

(Before abandoning your high blood pressure medication for a low-salt diet, be absolutely sure to get your doctor's approval.)

Cut Your Salt in Half

Whether you're salt sensitive or not—and regardless of your blood pressure level—cutting back on salt is usually a good idea, say scientists from Boston University's School of Medicine. Humans need only about a tenth of a teaspoon of salt per day. Yet most people take 2 teaspoons.

Simply by reducing your daily salt intake to 2,000 milligrams (or 1 teaspoon of salt) or less, you could lower your blood pressure several points in just a few weeks.

It's particularly important to keep your salt intake down if you're taking blood pressure medication, especially diuretics. Too much salt can actually undo the drug's pressure-lowering effect, increasing your need for higher doses of medications and thereby raising your risk of side effects.

Don't Go Cold Turkey

Salt can be addictive. If you try to give it up cold turkey, foods may taste flavorless at first. There are several ways around this dilemma. One is a little creative herb craft, replacing one flavor with others. At the same time, you'll notice that salt cravings usually diminish over time.

Scientists at the University of California at Davis School of Medicine illustrated it was so. They restricted the sodium intake of 43 people aged 25 to 49. Another group had no salt reduction. At the end of six months, both groups were served salted and unsalted soups, and were asked to mix the two until the soup reached the desired level of saltiness. The low-sodium subjects reduced their salting level by more than 50 percent, while the other group had virtually unchanged tastes.

Shake your salt habit slowly. For starters, remove the saltshaker from the counter or fill it with an herb combination— say, dill, paprika, and dried parsley. Later in this chapter, you'll find dozens of ways to use herbs and spices to add zing to your food without imparting any of salt's sting.

You might try one of the salt substitutes on the market if you have high blood pressure or take blood pressure medications, but use them sparingly. Salt substitutes get their salty flavor from po- tassium chloride rather than *sodium* chloride. Potassium chloride may interact with many medications, including some prescribed for hypertension, so it's important to consult a physician before switching to a salt substitute. For those with normal blood pres- sure, salt substitutes can be a good choice for cutting back on excess sodium in the diet.

Next, begin cutting salt in your recipes by two-thirds. Cook and bake using unsalted margarine and butter. Or use oil, which is salt-free. Switch to a low-sodium baking powder. Standard bak- ing powders contain a lot of sodium. A typical brand has 405 mil- ligrams per teaspoon. A low-sodium version can contain as little as 2 milligrams.

Sodium Cutbacks Are a Cinch

With all the brand-new "no-salt-added" products on the market today, you can prepare low-salt meals and snacks without surrendering a smack of flavor.

Take a cup of no-salt-added tomato sauce, for instance. Add it to your stew in lieu of the salted variety, and you'll be elimi- nating over 1,400 milligrams of sodium from your meal!

If life with green beans is just not bearable without salt, then try them with half the salt. Blend the unsalted variety (less than 10 milligrams of sodium per ½ cup) with the salted (442 milli- grams). No loss of flavor here, either.

So you say you really like that salty taste you get when biting into a peanut-butter cracker? Well, you can go halfway here, too. Regular peanut butter atop an unsalted cracker (or vice versa) can still have you yearning for more. The same is true of dip. Unsalted crackers can only enhance the flavor of the dip. The savings may seem small, but they add up in the long run.

Low-sodium cheeses can be a boon to the cook who wants to cut back without giving up cheese altogether. Eaten as a snack, low-sodium cheese may taste comparatively flat; but the difference is less noticeable when a mixture of low-sodium cheddar and Swiss is melted on homemade pizza or casseroles.

Become a Salt Sleuth

The fact is, most of our sodium is hidden—it's laced throughout processed foods, commercial baked goods, and fast foods. Surprisingly, even soft drinks can be notoriously high in the stuff. So even if you've virtuously replaced the salt in your shaker with herbs, you could still be overdosing on salt from that chicken soup you bought at the deli or the breakfast cereal you have each morning. A little vigilance is in order!

- Limit fast foods, processed foods, and convenience foods, unless they specifically indicate that they're low in sodium. A McDonald's Big Mac has 950 milligrams of sodium. A Burger King Whopper with cheese has 1,164 milligrams of sodium, which by itself nearly exceeds the recommended daily limit for those on sodium-restricted diets. A lot of the sodium comes from condiments and "extras," so tell the order-taker to "hold the cheese, mustard, ketchup, and pickle" on your hamburger—you'll cut the salt content of your favorite fast-food meal in half.
- Say "no thanks" to high-salt meats like bacon, ham, sausage, frankfurters, and luncheon meats.
- Try to avoid canned vegetables, which are higher in sodium than fresh or frozen.
- Read labels. Look for packaged products labeled "sodium-free" or "very low-sodium." Read ingredients closely. If salt or any other ingredient that contains sodium—such as monosodium glutamate—is among the first five ingredients, assume the product is high in sodium. Make another selection.

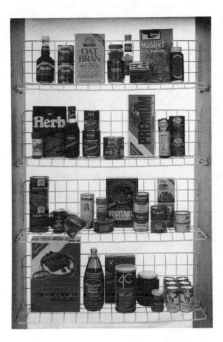

No-salt or low-salt products can help you keep your sodium intake to the recommended 2,000-milligrams-a-day level. Read labels with an eagle eye. If you spy the word "sodium" at the top of the ingredients list, pass up the product.

Rinse Canned Foods

Rinsing is one way to reduce the sodium content of food. In an experiment at Duke University Medical Center in North Carolina, chemists drained canned green beans and rinsed them under tap water for 1 minute. The sodium content of the beans dropped by 41 percent. Rinsing canned tuna for 1 minute cut sodium content by up to 79 percent.

When you're ready to cook your vegetables, microwave, steam, or sauté them—but don't cook them in salted water. Vegetables soak up sodium from the water.

Tasty Ways to Season without Salt

With some of the new flavor enhancers and some knowledge of how to use the right blends of herbs and spices, you'll never miss your saltshaker.

- Kikkoman makes "lite" soy sauce with 43 percent less salt—or 170 milligrams of sodium per teaspoon. The savings can really add up if you use it regularly.
- A dash of Angostura aromatic bitters can make up for that "missing something" when making gravies, sauces, or salad dressings. Would you believe that Angostura Bitters has been around since 1824? That's right—for over 160 years, and from the very beginning, according to a company spokesperson, it has been a no-salt-added flavor enhancer made from exotic herbs and spices. And it's all natural! It's a great condiment to pep up your no-sodium soups, casseroles, grain pilafs, and beverages. Because it is so versatile, you may find it in the condiment, gourmet, sodium-free, or cocktail-mix section of your supermarket.
- A bay leaf, a generous sprinkling of oregano, and a dash of garlic powder can spruce up a low-sodium spaghetti sauce if the taste doesn't suit you.
- Certain spices and fruits are natural for some foods. Curry, paprika, parsley, sage, tarragon, marjoram, oranges, cherries, and pineapple are well suited for chicken dishes. (Citrus, especially, provides the same kind of bite that salt does, without the sodium.) For fish, try bay leaf, marjoram, parsley, anise, dry mustard, green pepper, or ginger. For pork, try apple-sauce (there's no salt added there), apples, or sage.
- Sweet peppers, paprika, chili peppers, and ground chilies go well in soups and stews. Nutmeg can really highlight a vegetable dish. Don't be afraid to experiment with some bold flavors—coriander, cardamom, cumin, cloves, anise, and ginger. (Use small amounts, though, until you get acquainted with new seasonings and their potency.)
- When a recipe calls for bread crumbs and you haven't any no-salt bread, substitute no-salt dry cereal reduced to crumbs in a food mill, food processor, or electric blender.

- To pep up a meat loaf, use chopped onions, low-salt vegetable juice, and celery, including the tops.
- Low-salt or no-salt vegetable juice makes an excellent stock for a vegetable-beef soup.
- Allspice does wonders for low-salt cottage cheese and ricotta dishes.
- A few drops of lemon juice add zip to salt-free chicken, nut breads, and vegetables. Chicken soup without salt, for example, gets a nice lift from a bay leaf and a little lemon juice.
- Nut butters make great no-sodium spreads. As a change from butter on your morning toast, as a spread for sandwiches, and as a lift for your uncooked confections and baked goods, try the Westbrae line of sodium-free nut butters: almond, peanut, cashew, and sesame tahini. To make your snack low-sodium all the way, spread any one of these butters on no-salt brown-rice wafers.

A Guide to Low-Salt Entertaining

Chances are, many of your friends and relatives share your concern over salt. So you'll probably want to spare your dinner guests a big dose of sodium. Not too long ago, hosting low-sodium dinners and parties was a bit of a problem. To control the amount of salt, you had to make nearly everything from scratch. Today, you can get a healthy hand from the scores of no-salt and reduced-sodium products available in stores. Here's how to make every milligram count when setting the buffet table.

- Serve plenty of club soda and sparkling water. Most contain less than 50 milligrams of sodium per eight-ounce glass. Some have less than 10 milligrams. Read labels and choose brands that specify they're low-sodium or unsalted.
- Choose low-sodium vegetable-juice cocktails. A typical six-ounce serving has only 60 milligrams, compared with more than 500 milligrams for the salted kind.

- In the same vein, look for no-salt-added and reduced-sodium tomato juices.
- Zip up tomato-based drinks with a bit of horseradish, a pinch of cayenne, a few drops of hot-pepper sauce, a dash of bitters, or a generous squeeze of lemon or lime juice.
- Many low-sodium cheeses are making their way into dairy cases. The sodium savings can be impressive. For instance, choosing a 50 percent reduced-sodium cheddar can help you eliminate 130 milligrams of sodium per ½-ounce piece. A 75 percent reduced-sodium Swiss cheese can have as few as 26 milligrams per ½-ounce slice. Even regular Swiss cheese is a good idea, because Swiss is naturally lower in sodium than most other cheeses. It's got about half the sodium of cheddar or brick, for example, and only about one-fifth as much as blue cheese. Among other cheeses available in low- or reduced-sodium form are Gouda, Monterey Jack, Muenster, and Colby.
- No-salt and low-sodium crackers abound. Choose from wheat wafers, cracked-wheat wafers, bran wafers, rye wafers, melba rounds, melba toast, whole grain flatbreads, matzoh, sesame crackers, herbed wheat crackers, rice crackers, plain bread sticks, and sesame bread sticks. Other no-salt snack foods include potato chips, pretzels, corn chips, and tortilla chips.
- Popcorn is a perennial favorite. Make your own in a hot-air popper (to cut calories), then sprinkle it with one of your favorite herbs, no-salt herb blends, or cinnamon.
- Pick no-salt and reduced-salt pickles. Choose from kosher dills or spears, dill chips, and bread-and-butter chips.
- Add variety and color to a relish dish with no-salt hot cherry peppers or pickled sweet peppers.
- If you use olives, be aware that black olives usually contain about one-third the sodium of green ones. But also be aware that neither is low sodium.

- Set out no-salt ketchup, mayonnaise, chili sauce, spicy chutney, barbecue sauce, and green-peppercorn sauce. Use low-sodium soy sauce.
- Seek out no-sodium mustards. Salted mustards average 100 to 200 milligrams per tablespoon. Some varieties go as high as 445 milligrams. No-salt and low-sodium brands can slash that amount. Choose from hot, mild, sweet, sassy, coarse, smooth, and lemon sesame.
- Season your homemade dips with no-salt herb blends. There are a million (almost) to choose from. Try lemon herb, hot and spicy, Italian, Oriental, French, Mexican, and curry. Look for blends that are targeted especially for vegetables, fish, chicken, and steak.
- For fish and seafood dips, use no-salt clams, tuna, salmon, and sardines. If you've got salted varieties you'd like to use up, empty the cans into a colander, then rinse under cold water for a full minute. You'll wash away up to 90 percent of the sodium.
- When shopping, scan the shelves for salt-free vegetable dips, salsas, taco sauces, curry sauces, and sweet-and-sour sauces, often sold with dietetic foods.
- Serve unsalted roasted almonds, cashews, peanuts, sunflower seeds, and mixed nuts. An ounce of unsalted cashews, for instance, can have less than 10 milligrams of sodium; salted cashews can weigh in at around 180 milligrams.
- Buy peanuts roasted in their shell. Or roast chestnuts on an open fire (or in your oven). (Be sure to cut an X-shaped steam vent in each chestnut before heating, though, so they don't explode.)

Potassium and Calcium: Partners for Better Blood Pressure

You might want to go out today and hug a farmer. The prescription to keep your blood pressure down may be growing in his fields and orchards or grazing in his pastures right now.

Potassium, abundant in fresh fruits and vegetables, and calcium, found largely in many dairy products, may be science's latest dietary one-two punch in the fight against hypertension.

During the last few years, studies have uncovered what may be an important link between dietary calcium and potassium and blood pressure. Researchers have found that people whose diets are potassium-rich—vegetarians, for example—rarely develop hypertension even if they're genetically predisposed to the condition and don't control their salt intake.

Large-population surveys revealed the calcium connection: People with high blood pressure don't seem to get much calcium in the form of dairy products (and it's hard to get much without them). In one test, people who were mildly hypertensive and had lower levels of calcium in their blood experienced a moderate but consistent drop in blood pressure when they were given oral calcium supplements. The biggest improvement was seen in those people who had the lowest levels of calcium to start with. Studies like that are leading doctors to believe that there's far more to controlling blood pressure than cutting back on salt.

How the Minerals Work

The exact mechanisms by which the two essential nutrients regulate blood pressure continue to evade researchers. But both appear to help the body get rid of excess sodium and are involved in important functions that control the workings of your blood vessels and circulatory system.

"We need potassium to maintain proper body chemistry and to help compensate for the salty diets most of us eat today," explains Louis Tobian, M.D., head of hypertension programs at the University of Minnesota in Minneapolis. "Two or three servings of potassium-rich foods a day can help your body eliminate excess fluid and ease down your blood pressure."

And studies on calcium are promising for people with high blood pressure. Researchers have found that the more calcium in the diet, the lower the blood pressure.

Calcium may help the "salt sensitive."   Some studies indicated that some people might benefit from calcium and some might not—and that it may be possible to tell who's who. A 1986 study at New York Hospital–Cornell Medical Center showed that calcium works to lower blood pressure in the same people who are salt sensitive—that is, in those whose blood pressure rises in response to salt intake. And about 60 percent of people with high blood pressure seem to fit this criterion. Then, a 1988 study done at Purdue University found that, among other things, being older and having higher levels of parathyroid hormone made it more likely that calcium could have a pressure-lowering effect.

There are actually two possible explanations of how calcium might be able to reduce blood pressure levels, says Michael B. Zemel, Ph.D., associate professor of endocrinology and nutrition and food science at Wayne State University in Detroit. The first theory is simple: In salt-sensitive people, eating too much salt makes them retain water. That causes the amount of water in their blood vessels to go up, raising the pressure just like turning up the flow through a garden hose. That's why diuretics—drugs to make your body release water—lower blood pressure for some people. Calcium seems to help your kidneys release sodium and water, so you get a natural diuretic effect. (Dr. Zemel cautions that calcium is not a substitute for prescribed diuretics, and you should not stop taking any blood pressure medication on your own. Talk it over with your doctor first.)

The second is a little more complicated. It ties in the role of the parathyroid hormone, a link first identified in the Purdue study, says Dr. Zemel. Just as calcium helps salt-sensitive people excrete excess sodium, too much salt causes them to lose calcium from their blood. When this happens, the body responds by releasing parathyroid hormone plus another hormone derived from the vitamin D we get from food. Together, these two hormones pull calcium out of our bones and push it into the smooth muscle cells lining the blood vessels. Inside these cells, calcium forces the muscles to contract, which raises blood pressure like a hand squeezing tightly around a garden hose.

But eating a sufficient amount of calcium prevents the release of the parathyroid and vitamin D hormones, so no calcium is pushed into smooth muscle cells. Your blood vessels stay relaxed and blood pressure stays down.

Medicine That's Easy to Swallow

It's easy to work potassium and other helpful minerals into your menu. With a little ingeunity, you can build a diet around the foods supplying these nutrients.

Getting potassium isn't tough. "It's in almost everything," says Patricia Hausman, author of *The Calcium Bible*. It's abundant in foods that are good for you in other ways: fruits, vegetables, beans, fish, poultry, and lean cuts of meat.

Getting calcium is not quite as easy. Unfortunately, the foods that contain the most calcium tend to contain a fair amount of fat and sodium, too, which can spell trouble for hypertensives on fat-

and salt-controlled diets. Difficult does not mean impossible, however. There are plenty of low-fat, low-sodium dairy alternatives—and some calcium-rich foods that haven't even been near the dairy farm.

If you aren't hypertensive, by all means don't scratch milk and milk products off your shopping list. "For people to avoid milk because of sodium—unless you have hypertension—is not a good idea," says Leonard Braitman, Ph.D., a statistical consultant who worked on early calcium and hypertension studies. "For some people, like the lactose intolerant, it's not a good food. Many adults produce too little of the digestive enzyme needed to digest lactose, the primary sugar in milk. For other people, it's hard to beat. It's hard to make up your calcium intake with other foods. People should be aware that for people who have hypertension, sodium is a problem. But for others it's probably not."

Creative Cookery in Ten Easy Steps

Ready to start a diet that may last—and lengthen—a lifetime? The first rule of all good menu planning is to make a list. The two tables included in this chapter—"The Best Food Sources of Calcium" and "The Best Food Sources of Potassium"—can help you design your own hypertension diet. And here are a few tips to get you started.

1. Exercise your ingenuity. As you look over your list, envision new combinations of familiar foods: yogurt and bananas, salmon fillet with potatoes and broccoli, raisins and nuts. Imagine half a cantaloupe filled with a scoop of ice milk or ricotta cheese. Think about a summer cooler made in the blender from orange juice, bananas, and nonfat dry milk. You don't necessarily need a cookbook—experiment with your own combinations.

2. Browse through your cookbooks. Every home cookbook library is chock-full of recipes that are bypassed in lieu of family favorites. To rediscover combos that will help lower your blood pressure, start by consulting the indexes of your old standbys for the ingredients featured in the two tables. Then zero in on

The Best Food Sources of Calcium

Food	Portion	Calcium (mg)
Swiss cheese (LS)	2 oz.	544
Provolone cheese	2 oz.	428
Monterey Jack cheese	2 oz.	424
Yogurt, low-fat* (LS)	1 cup	415
Cheddar cheese	2 oz.	408
Muenster cheese	2 oz.	406
Colby cheese	2 oz.	388
Brick cheese	2 oz.	382
Sardines, Atlantic, drained solids*	3 oz.	372
American cheese	2 oz.	348
Ricotta cheese, part-skim	½ cup	337
Milk, skim* (LF,LS)	1 cup	302
Mozzarella cheese	2 oz.	294
Buttermilk*	1 cup	285
Limburger cheese	2 oz.	282
Ice milk, soft-serve* (LF,LS)	1 cup	274
Salmon, sockeye, drained solids* (LS)	3 oz.	271
Ice cream*	1 cup	176

dishes that are low in calories, fat, and sodium. (Many recipes will still work if you cut back on the amounts of salt and fat they call for.) You may discover new combinations of potassium- and calcium-rich foods that have been right under your nose for years. (If you reach a dead end, your local library probably has shelves of cookbooks to give you ideas, including many that feature recipes low in calories, fat, and sodium.)

3. Feature foods rich in both potassium and calcium.   Not only can you get potassium and calcium in the same dish, you can get them in the same food. A few of the foods

Food	Portion	Calcium (mg)
Ice milk* (LF,LS)	1 cup	176
Tofu (LF,LS)	3 oz.	174
Pizza, cheese	⅛ of 14" pie	144
Blackstrap molasses (LF)	1 Tbsp.	137
Soy flour, defatted	½ cup	120
Almonds* (LS)	¼ cup	100
Broccoli, cooked* (LF,LS)	½ cup	89
Soybeans, cooked* (LS)	½ cup	88
Parmesan cheese	1 Tbsp.	86
Collards, cooked (LF,LS)	½ cup	74
Dandelion greens, cooked	½ cup	74
Mustard greens, cooked (LF,LS)	½ cup	52
Kale, cooked (LF,LS)	½ cup	47
Broccoli, raw* (LF,LS)	1 cup	42
Chick-peas, cooked (LS)	½ cup	40

NOTE: If LF follows a food name, it indicates a low-fat food. If LS follows a food name, it indicates a low-sodium food.
*Food is also high in potassium.

that are high in both nutrients are: sardines, scallops, skim milk, broccoli, salmon, buttermilk, whole milk, soybeans, blackstrap molasses, navy beans, almonds, ice milk, and yogurt. Think of it: you can make a whole meal, from soup to nuts, using just a few of these double-duty foods.

4. Stock up on low-fat yogurt.   "It's a real bonanza food," says Arlene Caggiula, Ph.D., associate professor of nutrition at the University of Pittsburgh Graduate School of Public Health. Not only is yogurt low in fat and relatively low in sodium, it's high in calcium and potassium and can be used for everything

The Best Food Sources of Potassium

Food	Portion	Potassium (mg)
Potato, baked	1 medium	844
Avocado	½	602
Raisins	½ cup	545
Sardines, Atlantic, drained solids*	3 oz.	501
Flounder, baked	3 oz.	498
Orange juice	1 cup	496
Banana	1	471
Apricots, dried	¼ cup	448
Squash, winter, cooked	½ cup	445
Cantaloupe	¼ medium	413
Skim milk*	1 cup	406
Sweet potato, baked	1 medium	397
Salmon fillet, cooked*	3 oz.	378
Buttermilk*	1 cup	371
Whole milk*	1 cup	370
Round steak, trimmed of fat, broiled	3 oz.	352

from salad dressing to dessert. "Plain low-fat yogurt alone has 350 milligrams of potassium, and flavored low-fat yogurt has an average value of 450 milligrams," says Dr. Caggiula. "The best thing is that the low fat is even higher in potassium than regular yogurt." For high amounts of calcium, look for low-fat yogurt to which the manufacturer has added nonfat milk solids, suggests Hausman. It adds considerably more calcium and no more fat. She also suggests dressing up plain yogurt with potassium-rich foods such as frozen orange juice concentrate, raisins, sliced fresh fruit, or shredded raw vegetables. If you're not a yogurt fan, you can get all its benefits

Food	Portion	Potassium (mg)
Cod, baked	3 oz.	345
Great Northern beans, cooked	½ cup	344
Sirloin, trimmed of fat, broiled	3 oz.	342
Apricots, fresh	3	313
Beef liver, pan-fried	3 oz.	309
Haddock, fried	3 oz.	297
Pork, trimmed of fat, cooked	3 oz.	283
Tomato, raw	1	279
Leg of lamb, trimmed of fat, cooked	3 oz.	274
Turkey, light meat, roasted	3 oz.	259
Perch, fried	3 oz.	243
Tuna, drained solids	3 oz.	225
Chicken, light meat, roasted	3 oz.	210
Broccoli, cooked*	½ cup	127

*Food is also high in calcium.

by hiding it in blender shakes with fresh fruit and a sweetener, such as honey or aspartame, or in cold fruit soups.

5. Treat yourself to a Banana Smoothie.   You can add high-potassium and -calcium nonfat milk solids to dishes simply by adding nonfat dry milk. Two tablespoons of nonfat dry milk added to half a glass of skim milk boost the calcium from 150 to 255 milligrams. Add a banana, as Hausman does in her Banana Smoothie, and you've got a supercharged potassium-calcium breakfast.

Six Tips for Lactose Intolerance

In light of all the evidence showing calcium's blood-pressure-lowering effects, the best course for everyone is to try to get the 800 milligrams Recommended Dietary Allowance for calcium by eating lots of calcium-rich foods. But that can be harder if dairy foods leave you feeling gassy and bloated. But there are ways around lactose intolerance—an inability to properly digest the milk sugar, lactose. Try some of these proven alternatives:

1. Combine your dairy food with dinner. Lactose is easier to digest when mixed with other foods.
2. Eat smaller servings throughout the day. For instance, take small drinks of milk with each meal instead of downing an entire glass at once. Your body may be able to manage the lactose in installments.
3. Add cocoa to your low-fat milk. Although they still don't know why, researchers have found that cocoa makes milk more digestible.
4. Eat yogurt. Helpful bacteria in yogurt digest the lactose for you.
5. Select only cheeses aged six months or longer, like Swiss or cheddar. Aging breaks down most of the lactose in cheese.
6. Try liquid or tablet forms of lactase (available in drugstores), the milk-sugar-digesting enzyme that you're lacking. Or use milk that's made with lactase already added.

To make a Banana Smoothie, combine ¾ cup skim milk, ¼ cup nonfat dry milk, ½ tablespoon peanut butter, a very ripe banana, 1 tablespoon honey, and two ice cubes in a blender and process until smooth. One caution: though low in fat and sodium, this delicious drink is high in calories—282 per serving. If you're dieting, it's not the best snack or thirst quencher but a great and nutritious breakfast or lunch.

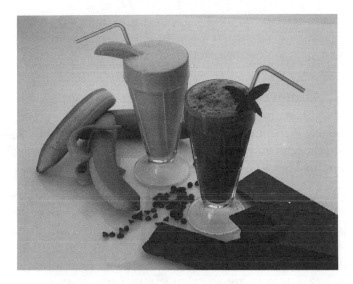

Which milkshake packs the blood-pressure-lowering punch? The one on the left. It's made with potassium-rich bananas and nonfat milk, a rich source of calcium. Both minerals help your body get rid of excess sodium and relax the blood vessels so blood can flow more easily.

When adding nonfat dry milk to milk products, use these proportions: 2 tablespoons milk powder to ½ cup milk, ¼ cup milk powder to 1 cup milk, 6 tablespoons milk powder to 1½ cups milk, and ½ cup milk powder to 2 cups milk.

6. Reach for ricotta. While cottage cheese and fruit may be a favorite summer lunch, you can substantially increase the amount of calcium in the meal by substituting ricotta. Though it also has more fat and calories than cottage cheese, ricotta has about 260 milligrams of calcium in ½ cup compared to only about 80 milligrams in cottage cheese. You can cut out some fat by using part-skim ricotta or by mixing it with low-fat cottage cheese. It's great served with high-potassium fruit, like apricots, too.

7. Toss together a stir-fry pizza. Make your own pizza dough—or buy it ready-made—but don't use the usual toppings.

Vegetables like carrots, onions, peppers, and broccoli (which is also high in calcium), either stir-fried in a bit of oil or steamed, take the place of tomato sauce. Top with part-skim mozzarella cheese and bake as usual.

8. Improvise with canned pink salmon. Salmon is high in potassium and calcium—because of the soft tiny bones you can eat—and mixes well with cheese and vegetables. Served hot with vegetables or as the star of a cold vegetable-pasta salad, salmon can become a staple of your blood pressure diet.

9. Use soy foods for a calcium payoff. If you have to restrict your dairy intake, soy foods such as tofu and some cooked beans can provide a modest amount of calcium. Tofu, in particular, can be used in place of cheese in many dishes. It has about 150 milligrams of calcium per 4-ounce serving. And tofu now can be processed to taste just like that summer treat, ice cream.

10. Enjoy shrimp, the special occasion star. Though high in cholesterol, shrimp is a fair source of calcium and a delicious ingredient of a vegetable stir-fry high in potassium.

Steaming Preserves Potassium

Don't plop that potato in boiling water. Steam your spuds instead. Swedish researchers discovered that when potatoes are boiled, up to 50 percent of their potassium leaches out into the cooking water. Worse, the potatoes can absorb sodium that has been added to the pot. In contrast, steamed potatoes lost as little as 3 percent of their potassium and gained practically no sodium. The researchers say that steaming also conserves potassium in carrots, beans, peas, and fish, all rich sources of this mineral.

Hit the Road for Lower Blood Pressure

Exercise might be just what the doctor ordered to help lower high blood pressure. Robert Cade, M.D., a University of Florida professor of medicine and the inventor of GatorAde, made this discovery when he got involved in his son's junior high science project.

The story goes like this: Dr. Cade's son designed a science project called "The Effect of Cardiovascular Response to Exercise in a Fat Old Man." The project called for the "fat old man"— his dad—to run daily for seven weeks and measure his blood pressure as he did so. Dr. Cade went along with this program and discovered that jogging produced a healthy decline in his mildly elevated blood pressure.

Since then, Dr. Cade has studied the effects of exercise on more than 400 people with high blood pressure, half of whom were taking medication for the disease. Ninety-six percent of them, he says, reduced their blood pressure significantly, fully 60 percent of those on medication went off it, and the rest reduced their dosage.

Other studies back up Dr. Cade's findings. In one, conducted by James Hagberg, Ph.D., a researcher at the National Institute on Aging, exercisers had an average 20-point drop in their systolic blood pressure and a 10-point drop in their diastolic pressure after completing an exercise program. That could make a big difference to someone with borderline high blood pressure!

Exercise works by forcing the blood vessels to open up (vasodilate), allowing blood pressure to come down, Dr. Cade says. "Even though it tends to go back up during exercise, it drops when exercise ends. Then when it goes back up, it docsn't go up as much."

Working out also helps make your heart more robust. A conditioned heart is more efficient; that is, it's able to pump out more blood with each beat. Moreover, a conditioned heart will have no difficulty pumping out more blood during exertion or an emergency, such as when you have to shovel snow off the driveway. An unconditioned heart may not be able to handle this sudden demand for more blood without serious straining. High blood pressure only compounds the problem and makes the heart work even harder.

Walking Is the Ideal Exercise

Doctors generally agree that to reduce blood pressure a workout has to be "aerobic." That is, it has to raise one's pulse to what's called the "target heart rate" for a half hour or so. (To figure out your target heart rate, subtract your age from 220, and then take 70 to 85 percent of that.)

Increasing your heart rate, however, doesn't mean you have to exercise to exhaustion. At the Institute for Aerobic Research in Dallas, a group of 64 men with mild hypertension—their diastolic pressure was between 90 and 104—undertook a program of conservative walk-jogging for 30 to 40 minutes a day, three times a week. Their progress was slow—it took four months—but eventually they reduced their systolic pressure by an average of 12.4 points and their diastolic pressure by nearly 7 points.

Regular walking is a good exercise for hypertension because unlike, say, a spirited game of one-on-one basketball, walking won't raise already-high blood pressure to dangerous levels. Yet walking gives the cardiovascular system a workout, promoting greater efficiency and lowering blood pressure. Also, walking regularly helps you lose weight, which also helps lower blood pressure.

Taking the First Step to Lower Blood Pressure

Walking is one of the simplest, most pleasant, and safest physical activities around. You might find that 30 minutes of walking is the easiest exercise to squeeze into your daily schedule. You can, for example, park several blocks away from the office and walk the rest of the way. Or you can cut your lunch hour short and walk for the remaining time.

Start slowly.   Phase in your walking program slowly—you're less likely to overdo it and quit before you've gained any benefits.

"We usually start people with walking a quarter of a mile briskly," says Dr. Cade. "Then we go up from there until a person can walk a mile briskly."

Don't worry if you don't even work up a sweat at first. Even walking at a slower pace can be beneficial, studies show. One study showed that a 40-minute walk, regardless of pace, significantly reduced both blood pressure and anxiety levels in people tested recently at the University of Massachusetts Center for Health and Fitness. The reductions lasted for at least 2 hours after the walking sessions were over and occurred whether the people walked at 35 percent, 50 percent, or 65 percent of their VO_2 Max (maximum aerobic capacity). The conclusion? Walking reduces blood pressure regardless of exercise intensity.

To begin your program, walk 5 minutes a day or one-fourth of a mile a day. As your endurance improves, slowly increase the time you walk until you can stride briskly for a half hour or so.

Wear comfortable shoes.   You don't have to buy special walking shoes if you've already got a good-fitting pair of running shoes. Shoes with plenty of cushioning in the heel are best for walking. Just don't use tennis or racquetball shoes, which are designed for quick changes in direction, not steady, rhythmic, one-directional impact.

Walk come rain or shine.   Try not to let bad weather get in the way of your walks. In extremely hot or cold weather, walk in a shopping mall, a museum, the hall of your apartment building, or around a track in a gym.

The Nautilus machine is a no-no.   If you are thinking of supplementing your walking program with a weight-lifting workout or a round on the Nautilus machine, don't. Weight lifting, or any kind of heavy tugging, pulling, or pushing, can constrict the blood vessels and overwork the heart. So if your blood pressure is elevated, leave the muscle building to the wrestlers— or check with your doctor.

In fact, it's a good idea to check with your doctor before embarking on any kind of regular exercise program.

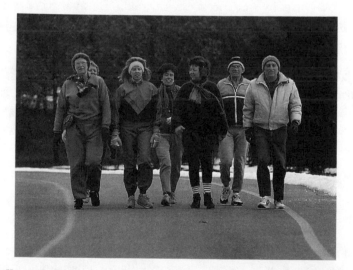

Walking helps lower blood pressure—but only if you keep at it. Don't let cold weather stop you. Bundle up in layers of clothing you can remove as you warm up. And take along some friends— the camaraderie of a shared experience takes the chill out of frosty weather.

Leave the Hand Weights at Home

Yes, carrying hand weights can substantially boost the oxygen demands and hence calorie-burning and fitness-building potential aspects of aerobic exercise. That's the good news.

But with the boost may come one small bust—a potentially dangerous rise in blood pressure for some people, report researchers from the University of Florida. Their study measured the effects of carrying hand weights (of either 1 or 3 pounds) on 12 healthy volunteers (aged 25 to 38) as they walked at varying speeds on a treadmill. At all workloads, energy requirements increased in direct response to the amount of weight carried—good for weight loss and cardiovascular endurance. Unfortunately, blood pressure also increased, and at a rate disproportionate to increases in energy output. At a workload of 75 percent of maximum *with* hand weights, for example, systolic blood pressures of the volunteers averaged 9 points higher than when that same 75 percent workload was achieved without weights.

Apparently, additional exercise on the smaller muscles in your arms can raise your blood pressure, sometimes to dangerous levels.

For most exercisers, such an increase poses no danger, say the researchers. But for people with high blood pressure or other cardiovascular quirks, the increase could be an unhealthy one. Play it safe and check with your doctor if you're thinking of adding hand weights to your workout.

Explore a Different Path

If your walking program has become too routine, consider these ways to maintain your interest and beat boredom.

The camera walk. Ever walk down the street with a

photographer? In the middle of a conversation you suddenly realize your companion is 20 feet behind you, taking a picture of an unusual sign, a flower, an icicle—or maybe of you. Things you've seen a thousand times but never really looked at. The point is, take a camera on your next walk—you'll be amazed how new objects, patterns, colors, and ideas come into focus.

The kid walk.   There's no way to predict what will interest a child. Here's a report filed by a grown-up who recently learned a walking lesson from a 14-month-old toddler.

"We were walking through a park, and I was pointing out all the things I thought she'd like—squirrels, dogs, trees. She wasn't too interested. Suddenly, she stopped. She stared downward, with a look of utter fascination. She reached down to the sidewalk and picked up—solemnly, with a face full of awe, then holding it up to me like a sacred offering—the itty-bittiest crushed scrap of a fragment of a brown leaf. I looked at small things differently after that."

The dog walk.   Pets provide company and affection—in fact, some therapists recommend them as remedies for depression and loneliness. But owning a dog has the added advantage of forcing you to get frequent exercise, which is not necessarily the case with a cat or a goldfish. Plus, walking a dog is a terrific way to make new friends, both canine and human.

The morning walk.   This kind of walk is in a class by itself. The world is different in the morning. Normally busy city streets are tranquil canyons that echo the cries of swooping birds. Meanwhile, country roads shimmer as the sun's rays illuminate the dew. You'll probably find a steady walking partner or two. And the air has that crisp, clear quality that's delightfully refreshing.

The Thoreau walk.   "I frequently tramped eight or ten miles through the deepest snow to keep an appointment with a beech tree, or a yellow birch, or an old acquaintance among the pines," wrote the nineteenth-century naturalist Henry David Thoreau. You, too, can make friends with the trees—and the flowers and the birds—with the help of a good guidebook.

"When you identify a tree," says Deborah Brien, a historian

and folklorist who teaches workshops on seasonal traditions for the Arnold Arboretum of Harvard University, the Cambridge Center for Adult Education, and the Massachusetts Audubon Society, ''it really does become your friend. And it gives you something important—oxygen. Everytime you pass it, you think, 'Hello! I know you! You're a little different today.' ''

What? Even if you live in the heart of the city, you may be surrounded by nature. (Why do you think they call it an ''urban jungle?'') The streets and buildings of New York City, for example, are home to not only pigeons and people, but also sparrows, gulls, falcons, and nighthawks, says Starr Saphir, a director of the New York City Audubon Society, who leads nature walks in the Big Apple. What's more, city parks are often teeming with wildlife, says Saphir. In Central Park, a keen-eyed birder could spot some 250 kinds of birds, including the North American songbirds. Not to mention fish, turtles, snakes, raccoons, and squirrels. Plus wild flowers. And of course, trees.

The Best Stress-Busters for a Healthier Heart

Stress hits us every day in big and little ways. We're overcharged on the electric bill. We have a fender bender on the way to work. The kid next door sets off firecrackers all evening. These everyday stresses prompt your body to pump out adrenaline, a powerful hormone that makes your heart pump faster and your blood vessels narrow. As a result, your blood pressure shoots up when you're under stress.

No one is sure whether chronic stress is responsible for hypertension. Some evidence indicates that people with high blood pressure have higher levels of adrenaline circulating in their blood than people with normal blood pressure do.

"It just makes sense to find ways to manage stress and give yourself a break from the constant bombardment of adrenaline," says Marvin Moser, M.D., clinical professor of medicine, Yale University School of Medicine, and author of *How to Control High Blood Pressure without Drugs*.

Select Your Rx for Stress Control

Doctors often prescribe various methods of stress control—relaxation techniques, biofeedback, and deep breathing, to name a few. These methods not only lower blood pressure for the time they're practiced, but also reduce tension—and blood pressure—around the clock.

Anything that relaxes you, makes you feel more in control, and helps your cares fade away can help break the stress-hypertension cycle. You might try a half hour of hand-sanding furniture or painting with watercolors. You can soak in a hot tub laced with aromatic mineral salts. Or you can try one of the following on-the-spot ways to defuse mental stress.

Choose the stress-coping technique that most appeals to you, because they all help to keep a lid on blood pressure. Better yet, try several techniques. Remember—every little bit of pressure lowering helps!

Relax from head to toe.   Progressive muscle relaxation is a proven technique for relieving stress. Sit or lie in a comfortable position, then tense and relax the muscles of your body, one muscle group at a time. Start by clenching your fists for 3 or 4 seconds, concentrating on how the tension feels, then relax your hand muscles, letting go of the tension.

Try this tensing/relaxing sequence for all major muscles—those in your neck, shoulders, back, arms, abdomen, buttocks, thighs, calves, and feet. Ideally, you'll learn to relax these muscles without tensing them first. Try this exercise for 10 minutes, twice a day.

Learn to handle anger.   Researchers have found that either holding anger in or blowing your top without trying to solve a problem can lead to an immediate (and possibly prolonged) rise in blood pressure.

On the other hand, people who handle their anger with what is called ''reflective coping'' seem to have lower blood pressure. The idea behind reflective coping is simple: You try to identify what stirs you up and why, and what happens when you react the way you do.

You might try keeping a diary of your anger—what sets you off and how you react. Then start developing new, more constructive ways to deal with your anger. Next time you get ticked off when someone cuts you off in traffic, you can take a deep breath, count to ten, and remind yourself it isn't worth an elevated blood pressure.

Learning how to handle the anger on the home front is especially important. One study found that when communication is a problem in families, everyone's blood pressure goes up.

So try a little reflective coping with your partner. Wait for your anger to subside and then rationally discuss the conflict. Don't blame each other. When you blame someone, you attack his self-worth and invite a counterattack. Instead of dwelling on criticism and negative judgments, focus on positive ways to solve the problem.

Pet your dog.   Or your rabbit. Or your cat. Any animal that's soft and cuddly. Researchers have found that when you pet a soft and cuddly animal, you lower your blood pressure. When you stroke your pet, it seems your voice becomes more gentle and your speech slows.

Some experts believe that the slower you speak, the more you pause for breath, the more you "downshift" your body and put your blood pressure in lower gear. "The minute you start talking to and petting your dog, your blood pressure goes down and stays down during the interaction," says Aline Halstead Kidd, Ph.D., professor of psychology at Mills College in Oakland, California. "The point is, human-to-human interactions make certain demands. A pet allows you to interact with another living being that makes no demands and loves you without regards to anything."

Watch the clouds roll by.   Turn your gaze to the birds circling the sky. Or the ripples of waves breaking on the river bank or flames crackling in a fireplace. "When you turn your attention to the natural environment, you are forced to look and listen instead of thinking and worrying," says psychiatrist Aaron Katcher, M.D., of the University of Pennsylvania. "Shutting off this worrisome internal dialogue is a great way to control tension and lower blood pressure." Based on studies of other relaxation techniques,

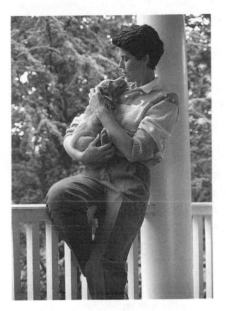

*Your dog—or your cat—
may be your blood
pressure's best friend.
Studies show that the
blood pressure of people
temporarily dropped
when they talked to or
petted a dog. But the
pet has to be one you
are familiar with; an
unfamiliar pooch could
make your blood
pressure rise.*

Dr. Katcher believes that doing any of these things for 15 minutes twice a day may be an effective treatment for some people with mild hypertension.

Smell a slice of apple pie.   Preliminary research suggests that certain scents—particularly spiced apple—may nearly double any blood-pressure-lowering benefits of quiet relaxation. One theory is that the smell of apple pie can trigger pleasant associations with holidays. The research is too limited to conclude that any given odor will nudge your own blood pressure down. But if you want to test the notion, try a fragrance you find particularly appealing. (See the chapter "Checking Your Blood Pressure.")

Plant a petunia.   Plant a few seeds, and you'll grow more than just zucchini in your garden. That's right. Along with flowers and vegetables, gardening can lead to stress resistance and lower your blood pressure.

When you escape from your revved-up, high-tech world and take refuge in the primitive peace of your garden, experts say you can rejuvenate your body and soul in scientifically measurable ways.

One leading researcher who has measured physiological responses to green, living things is Roger Ulrich, Ph.D., associate professor of geography at the University of Delaware and an expert in plant/people relationships.

Dr. Ulrich's studies showed that fairly substantial physiological and emotional changes occurred when people were exposed to plants. Their blood pressure lowered, their muscles loosened, and their heart rate slowed.

Researchers in the Netherlands unearthed a similar discovery. They found that people who lovingly tend their plants have significantly fewer heart attacks than those who never stop to smell—or grow—the roses. Gardening lowers blood pressure and increases the body's resistance to stress, the researchers concluded.

Listen to music.   Music can bring on a relaxation response similar to the one you might achieve by practicing meditation! Music that approximates your own heartbeat and breathing rate tends to be more relaxing, experts say. That's music with a rhythm of about 1 beat per second.

Parts of certain classical pieces come closest to fitting that description, particularly the slow second movements of some baroque pieces by Bach, Handel, and Telemann. But you're the best judge of whether music is relaxing to you. Whatever you find soothing, treat yourself to a relaxing music break today.

Cut back on caffeine.   If you drink a caffeinated beverage like coffee, tea, or cola while you're under stress, your blood pressure may rise. A study by Gwendolyn A. Pincomb, Ph.D., and other researchers in the Behavioral Sciences Laboratory of the Oklahoma City Veterans Administration Medical Center found that drinking a caffeinated beverage and preparing for exams raised blood pressure considerably higher than did either consuming caffeine or studying in themselves. What's more, the effect of the caffeine lingers, raising average blood pressure for at least two hours. This effect may become more pronounced as you get older, since many people's blood vessels tend to become less flexible with age.

So people who have high blood pressure (or who are at risk for high blood pressure) should be aware that too much caffeine may put even more pressure on already-stressed blood vessels.

If drinking coffee in an already stressful situation seems to jack up your blood pressure or your anxiety level, it makes sense to cut back on both coffee and stress. For starters, switch to decaffeinated coffee. In taste tests of unlabeled brews, coffee drinkers rarely distinguish between decaffeinated and regular. Or try herbal tea. With so many perk-me-up flavors around, you're sure to find at least two or three you really like.

Enjoy a good laugh.   A hearty laugh causes a small, temporary decrease in blood pressure. But even more important, laughter is a great way to relieve stress and anger. Go to a funny movie. Spend time with people who make you laugh, not complainers or argumentative types. The long-term effects of laughter on blood pressure are unknown, but certainly there are no negative side effects to laughing.

Be a happy person.   A study at New York Hospital–Cornell University Medical Center showed that different emotions play a very specific role in determining how high or low your blood pressure may go.

When testing unmedicated hypertensive patients around the clock with high-tech monitors, researchers found that happiness caused systolic blood pressure to drop, while anxiety caused diastolic pressure to rise. They also found that blood pressure changes were directly related to emotional intensity, so that the happier a person felt, the more the systolic pressure fell. Conversely, the more anxiety a person experienced, the higher the diastolic pressure rose.

Researchers also discovered that anxiety experienced outside the home makes blood pressure increase significantly more than anxiety experienced inside the home. The lesson in all this could be summed up as follows: Don't worry, be happy—but if you must worry, do it at home.

Turn On the Relaxation Response

Whether you tip over a canoe, debut as Othello at the Metropolitan Opera, or find yourself trapped in a traffic snare, your body reacts roughly the same: with the fight-or-flight response to stress that you inherited from your early ancestors. Heart rate, blood pressure, and breathing rate leap. Muscles tense. Adrenal glands work overtime. This reaction is appropriate for modern equivalents of the occasional tiger hunt, but you don't need all that adrenaline for most of life's everyday stressful challenges.

If a full-blown stress reaction becomes part of your routine, it may usher in a host of stress-induced physical ailments, such as high blood pressure.

Wouldn't it be great to be able to invoke the complete opposite response or to cut the fight-or-flight response off at the pass, unless you really need it?

Well, you can. In his famous book *The Relaxation Response,* Herbert Benson, M.D., introduced Americans to the flip side of the stress response. He dubbed it the "Relaxation Response." And it doesn't occur naturally. You have to learn to summon it with regular sessions of serene solitude.

The Relaxation Response is essentially a form of meditation, and as such it's not entirely new. It's been an integral part of centuries-old religious rituals. What Dr. Benson did was to study these rituals and devise a simplified way to achieve the same end: flicking the switch that turns off tension and, like meditation, turns on physical and mental peace. Here's Dr. Benson's method: to practice the technique, find a quiet environment, free of distractions. If you must, hang a "Do Not Disturb" sign on the door.

1. Choose a soothing or neutral word or phrase—a "mantra"—to focus on. Dr. Benson recommends "one," but you may prefer something else, like "love" or "peace." Whatever your choice, stick with it, because you'll eventually come to associate the word with calming effects.
2. Sit upright in a comfortable postion, with your hands resting naturally in your lap.
3. Gently close your eyes.
4. Take a few moments to relax your muscles, beginning at your feet and working up to your face. Keep them relaxed.

The Do-It-Yourself Stress Test

You can feel perfectly calm and still have hypertension, or feel like a nervous wreck and have normal blood pressure. But most people react to stress with at least a temporary rise in blood pressure. To find out if stress is boosting your blood pressure, test yourself. Buy a home blood-pressure monitor and have it calibrated by your physician or pharmacist. (Otherwise, it may be off by as much as 30 points.) Your doctor can show you the proper technique for taking your pressure. Then take your blood pressure before, during, and after a stressful activity. This way you'll know if the stressful event is affecting your blood pressure and whether you should avoid it. Good news: Not all stressful or exciting situations have an effect.

And while you're at it, check your spouse's pressure, too. You've probably heard that husbands and wives start looking alike after several years of marriage, but researchers have discovered an even stranger phenomenon: The longer two people are married, the more similar their blood pressure levels become.

The researchers who conducted the study suggest that this mimicking effect could have something to do with shared stress or other emotional factors. "Communication, particularly handling conflict and expressing emotions, may affect both spouses' blood pressure levels," says one. So if you find that your blood pressure is climbing, check your spouse's blood pressure, too. If you're both in your sixties, this study predicts that your blood pressures will be only a point or so apart.

5.   Breathe naturally through your nose and become aware of your breathing. Working with the slow, natural rhythm of your breathing, repeat your focus word silently on every exhale.

6. Maintain a passive attitude. Don't worry about whether or not you're achieving a state of deep relaxation. Let relaxation come to you. If distracting thoughts enter your mind, try not to dwell on them. Instead, return to your word. Dr. Benson emphasizes that this passive attitude is perhaps the most important element in bringing on the Relaxation Response.

7. Continue for 10 to 20 minutes. You may open your eyes to check the time, but don't use an alarm clock. After you finish, sit quietly with your eyes closed for a few moments. Then open your eyes and sit still for a few more minutes before you stand up.

The many healthful benefits of the Relaxation Response continue for as long as you keep practicing the method regularly. Dr. Benson and others have shown that it counteracts the stress response. It decreases blood pressure, lowers heart and respiration rates, decreases blood flow to the muscles, and slows body metabolism. If you have high blood pressure, it might drop to normal without drugs. You may find that you don't fly off the handle or get anxious quite as easily. You'll probably calm down.

This doesn't mean regularly practicing the Relaxation Response will prevent you from experiencing the fight-or-flight response when it's warranted. But you'll probably be more calm in the face of those everyday stressors, the hassles that *un*necessarily trigger on the fight-or-flight response.

What You Need to Know about Blood Pressure Drugs

Do you need medication to lower your blood pressure?

Maybe you do; maybe you don't. Doctors at Boston University Medical Center say that generally, you should first try nondrug therapies—salt restriction, weight loss, exercise, and stress management—if you have a diastolic pressure of 90 to 95. After 3 or 4 weeks of such therapies, your doctor should be able to tell whether or not they're working. If not, then drug treatment may be appropriate. Some people with a diastolic pressure of 96 to 99 can also try a nondrug therapy—if they're willing to work hard. Usually those at or above a diastolic pressure of 100 should be treated with medication.

As for people with moderate to severe hypertension—the 30 percent who have diastolic pressure above 104—they have little choice but to take anti-hypertensive drugs to control their disease. The higher blood pressure levels are just too risky to let them go unchecked. Consider that if you have a high blood pressure problem and are between the ages of of 45 and 74, you're three times more likely to have a heart attack and seven times more likely to have a stroke than someone with normal blood pressure.

Given these facts, anti-hypertensive drugs are "lifesavers in that they prevent the long-term complications that come with high blood pressure," says Norman M. Kaplan., M.D., head of the hypertension section at the University of Texas Southwestern Medical School in Dallas.

How Drugs Lower Pressure

Drugs are usually prescribed after diet therapy has been tried. As you'll recall from earlier chapters, high blood pressure occurs when blood vessels are overfilled and tight, like a thin hose hooked to a water faucet that's opened full force. If you're prescribed a medication to control your blood pressure, you'll be given one of three main types of drugs—a diuretic, a sympathetic nervous inhibitor, or a vasodilator. All three drugs cause the pressure to drop and the blood to flow more easily.

Diuretics are generally tried first. Diuretics reduce blood pressure by flushing out water and sodium, thereby reducing the load on the heart and blood vessels.

The next step is to try a sympathetic inhibitor. This type of drug, which includes the beta-blockers, causes the nerves surrounding the blood vessels to stop the flow of adrenaline, thereby widening the vessels.

The vasodilators act directly on the blood vessel to dilate it, much the same as you would loosen a belt after a big meal.

One in two people won't need more than a diuretic; the other may need more than one drug. Complicating matters is the fact that all three categories of drugs work differently in different people. "We would like to be able to predict which drugs will work," says Herbert Langford, M.D., of the University of Mississippi Medical School in Jackson, "but for now we have to operate according to trial and error."

What this means is that your doctor might have to prescribe several drugs or combinations of drugs before he finds the one that is right for you. So don't be discouraged if you're switched from medication to medication.

The Downside to Drugs

Unfortunately, up to one-half of the people who are supposed to take blood pressure medications simply don't. No wonder! The side effects can be bothersome and serious. All three types can cause dizziness, stomach upset, ulcers, depression, diarrhea, dry mouth, sexual dysfunction, slowed heart rate, or mineral depletion.

Take diuretics, for example. Along with all that water and sodium these drugs drain away, they also flush away certain essential minerals, namely potassium, magnesium, and calcium.

Medications and exercise don't mix.   Diuretics are also associated with digestive problems and can even undo the benefits of a good workout, studies suggest.

That's a problem, because exercise is usually another part of the anti-hypertension prescription. A team of doctors at Veterans Administration Hospital in Albuquerque reviewed 71 studies on the effects of anti-hypertensive drugs on exercise performance in people without coronary heart diseases. They found that the two most commonly used classes of drugs—beta-blockers (Inderal, Lopressor, Tenormin, Blocadren, and Corgard) and diuretics—cut endurance and work capacity during exercise.

In a similar study conducted by the University of Vermont School of Medicine involving 30 hypertensives, 10 patients were placed on the beta-blocker propranolol, 10 others were placed on another beta-blocker, metoprolol, and another 10 took a placebo (an inactive pill). Those on propranolol apparently reaped no benefits from 10 weeks of strenuous exercise. (These benefits usually include lowered blood pressure and improved cardiovascular fitness.) The researchers say that even though propranolol itself effectively lowers blood pressure, the drug apparently blocks the additional blood-pressure-lowering effects of regular workouts.

If you are exercising regularly and taking beta-blockers to control your blood pressure, ask your doctor about alternative drugs. The Veterans Administration doctors report that the calcium channel blockers (Procardia, Cardizem), the alpha antagonists (Minipress, Catapres, Tenex), the alpha-blockers (Normodyne, Trandate), or the converting enzyme inhibitors (Captone, Vasotec) are less likely to interfere with your workouts.

Additionally, researchers at the University of Vermont found that in the group who took metoprolol, the cardiovascular benefits of exercise were not as blunted as observed in the group that took propranolol.

A problem for men.   There's more to the downside of beta-blockers. In men, these drugs have also been shown to interfere with sex drive and performance.

"It's a problem of major proportion," Sydney Croog, Ph.D., professor of behavioral sciences and community health at the University of Connecticut Health Center, told *Men's Health* newsletter. "Because of side effects of anti-hypertensive drugs, many men view the treatment of high blood pressure as worse than the disease. And for legitimate reasons. Many drugs presently being used for controlling hypertension can have very discouraging effects, not just on sexual performance but on intellectual performance, emotions, and energy levels as well."

To assess the extent of the sexual problems associated with blood pressure drugs, Dr. Croog conducted a nationwide survey. "We asked men to rate on a scale of 1 to 5 the degree to which they had been distressed by a decrease in sexual interest, problems with achieving an erection, problems with maintaining an erection, or problems with ejaculations. We found that fully 60 percent of men taking medication for hypertension reported some degree of sexual dysfunction within the previous month. This compared with only 44 percent of hypertensives not on medication."

Considering that many closet hypertensives do not even see their doctors in the first place for fear they'll need anti-hypertensive medication, "you begin to see the magnitude of the problem," Dr. Croog said. "Men need to be made aware that not all medications have the same effects on their sex lives. Most of all, there has to be better communication between doctors and patients about the problem. Frequently men will simply discontinue taking a medication instead of discussing sexual problems and treatment alternatives."

Some drugs put the squeeze on your heart. Some drugs decrease blood pressure while *increasing* blood cholesterol. So some people who take these drugs have trouble getting their cholesterol down. (Researchers believe that for every 1 percent increase in blood cholesterol, heart attack risk goes up 2 percent.) As a result, many high blood pressure sufferers are also treated with cholesterol-lowering drugs. Such medications are often very expensive and frequently have unpleasant side effects of their own. For some people, the drugs are essential because of a genetic predisposition, but for others, high cholesterol may have been triggered by their blood pressure pills.

If your doctor wants to put you on blood pressure medicine, check to make sure that it doesn't increase cholesterol. If you take any blood pressure medication that raises cholesterol, have a complete blood cholesterol profile test, showing total cholesterol, high-density lipoprotein (HDL), low-density lipoprotein (LDL), and HDL/LDL ratio. And repeat the tests at a later date to make sure your cholesterol level has not increased. (In some cities, you can have these tests taken at no charge if you donate blood to the Red Cross.) If your cholesterol does go up, read on.

New Drugs Minus the Complications

Luckily, a number of effective anti-hypertensive drugs exist which don't increase cholesterol. These include the calcium channel blockers (Adalat, Calan, Cardizem, Isoptin, and Procardia), the ACE inhibitors (Capoten, Vasotec, and Prinivil), the vasodilator Apresoline, and the alpha-blocker prazosin (Minipress).

ACE inhibitors are revolutionizing the treatment of hypertension because they don't cause the fatigue, forgetfulness, sexual side effects, or depression that are common with beta-blockers and some other anti-hypertensive medications. But they have to be used very carefully. If your kidney function is not normal, they may be quite toxic. Thus, before taking these drugs, make sure the doctor does a creatinine clearance test. And avoid potassium-containing salt substitutes while taking the ACE inhibitors. With these drugs, too much potassium can be just as dangerous as too little.

On the horizon, Minipress looms as a healthful alternative. This drug actually appears to *decrease* cholesterol levels. Minipress may also turn out to be useful for prostate problems. According to preliminary reports, Minipress relaxes the smooth muscle in the prostate that makes urination difficult for some men with prostate problems. Minipress may thus help postpone the need for prostate surgery in susceptible men. This could be an important boon to the millions of older men who experience diminished urine flow due to enlargement of the prostate gland.

If you have high blood pressure and need to take medication, discuss the cholesterol issue with your doctor. Know your options and make sure you keep track of your own cholesterol levels.

Drugs that won't lower your sex drive.   There are a variety of other drugs that let a man have healthy blood pressure and a robust libido, too.

Doctors now know that one is captopril. Dr. Croog, along with other researchers at the University of Connecticut Health Center, Boston University, and 28 other institutes across the country, recently conducted a double-blind, controlled, randomized study comparing the sexual effects of three of the most common blood pressure medications prescribed today: captopril, propranolol, and methyldopa. Captopril emerged the clear winner, as the following results show:

- Patients treated with captopril experienced fewer sexual problems than those treated with methyldopa or propranolol.
- Interest in sex did not lessen with captopril but did decrease with methyldopa and propranolol.
- The ability to maintain an erection did not change with captopril but did diminish with the other two drugs.
- Negative effects on sexuality were found to be greatest in men 51 years or older who were taking methyldopa or propranolol plus a diuretic.

The results "point to the need for hypertensive patients to openly discuss their sexual symptoms and other possible drug side

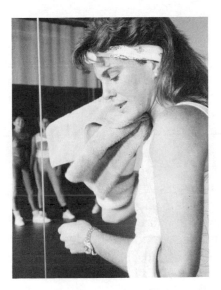

Some blood pressure medications can block the cardiovascular effects of your workout. If you have mild hypertension, you may be able to make dietary and lifestyle changes so you can eliminate drugs or reduce your dosage. Talk to your doctor.

effects with their doctors. Then, if needed, the physician can select an appropriate medication for that patient," says Dr. Croog.

Stick to the Treatment Plan

Once you and your doctor find the right medication, take drugs according to schedule—*especially* when you feel well. Many people stop taking their drugs when they feel good and trigger a potentially dangerous relapse of high blood pressure. Should you forget to take your medication for a couple of days, don't try to make up for it by taking the pills you missed. Instead, just resume taking them according to the schedule your doctor outlined.

Be sure that you ask your doctor to explain all the side effects associated with your drug therapy. So if you feel bad, you'll know whether you should contact your doctor. Side effects are a sign that your medication should be changed. In any case, anyone who has high blood pressure should see his doctor periodically to make sure it hasn't gotten worse. (Maybe he'll tell you you've improved!)

How to Say Bye-Bye to Blood Pressure Pills

Even if you've been taking blood pressure medicine for years, it's worth a try to make lifestyle changes that help control blood pressure without drugs. Such changes might make it possible for you to stop or reduce your medication in the future.

Is Your Blood Pressure Too Low?

For some people, the problem isn't high blood pressure but rather *low* blood pressure (called hypotension). They may experience a dizzy spell—or even faint—if they stand up too fast. Other possible symptoms include light-headedness, weakness, fatigue, or headaches.

Typically defined as a consistent fall of more than 20 mm/Hg systolic pressure when measured after 1 minute of standing, hypotension was once believed to afflict nearly as many elderly people as its opposite condition, hypertension. But over the last few years studies have shown that among healthy, nonmedicated elderly people, the rate of hypotension is only about 6 percent and does not increase with age after 55.

In many cases, apparently, hypotension is caused by the medications people take for hypertension, such as diuretics. Alcohol, as well as certain heart medications, tranquilizers, and antidepressants, has also been implicated.

If appropriate, and if you believe medication is causing symptoms associated with hypotension, you may need to ask your doctor to change a prescription. If that can't be done, though, there are still some other ways to alleviate this condition.

Try a Tight Squeeze

Studies have shown that relatively simple physical actions that momentarily elevate blood pressure can offset

As we mentioned previously, 70 percent of all hypertensives whose diastolic pressure falls between 90 and 104 (this range is called "mild hypertension") have the option of taking the medication or first trying one of the nondrug therapies. And considering the increasing cost of drugs and the possible side effects, it's worth a try.

hypotension. An isometric exercise like squeezing a handgrip before getting up, for example, can increase blood pressure enough to counter the momentary dip it takes upon standing.

Do Some Mental Math

More amazing, the researchers who documented the handgrip effect found that doing complex mental arithmetic (try counting backward from 100 by sevens as fast as you can) elevated blood pressure and offset hypotension even better than physical activity.

Eat Smaller, More Frequent Meals

If you typically experience hypotension after meals, try eating smaller, more frequent meals throughout the day. Also, find out how much salt and fluid intake your doctor recommends. Cutting back on salt and fluid may contribute to hypotension.

Sleep on a Slant

The way you sleep may also be important in helping control hypotension. Try sleeping with the head end of your bed elevated 8 to 12 inches higher than the foot end (use cement building blocks). When you get up in the morning, sit up slowly and dangle your feet over the edge of the bed for a few moments before standing.

If you are in this mild hypertension group, studies show that you may be able to drop your pressure without drugs. One of these studies, conducted at the University of Medicine and Dentistry of New Jersey, involved 86 men (average age of 57) whose resting diastolic blood presure (the second number of your blood pressure reading) was 95 to 105. The men were broken into two groups for three months of different treatments.

In one group, the men were given either the blood-pressure-lowering drug propranolol twice daily or two placebo pills that looked like propranolol, but that contained no active drug. The men in the other group got no pills at all. Instead, they exercised; modified their intake of salt, fat, and alcoholic beverages; and attended weekly stress-management sessions. (The men in the drug-or-placebo group received no such counseling and made no changes in their diet or exercise habits.)

By study's end, the men who had exercised, improved their diets, and reduced their stress had an average blood pressure reduction of nearly 13 points compared with only 8 points for those on drug therapy.

The beauty of this is that nondrug techniques double as disease *prevention* for people who are susceptible to high blood pressure but are still healthy. But remember: Your physician should guide you, regardless of the therapy you may prefer.

At this point, there's no way to say with any certainty whether or not people with more-severe hypertension will be able to achieve total control of their condition with a diet and exercise program. But experts feel that even for people with high hypertension, adopting the right diet and exercise program may allow them to lower their drug dosage and possibly even become drug-free.

Eight Weeks to Lifetime Blood Pressure Control

Throughout this book, you have learned that if you're one of the millions of Americans with high blood pressure, the future is bright. You've learned that you need not be sentenced to a lifetime of medication and that you don't have to eat bland meals that make your taste buds scream for just one pickle.

You've also read that researchers have been hot on the trail of lifestyle treatments that can lower blood pressure without drugs and without taking the pleasure out of life. They say that if your diastolic pressure (the second number) is between 85 and 104 (mild hypertension), you stand a good chance of lowering your blood pressure enough to get off medication entirely—or never having to start. And even if your numbers are higher, you may be able to cut way back on medication. All of this without embracing the austere existence of a monk.

The best of these nondrug approaches have been distilled into the following eight-week program. It's doctor-approved and based on the most effective anti-hypertension strategies discussed in earlier chapters.

The program goes slow and easy because sudden lifestyle changes are discouraging and rarely last. The idea is to phase in a few small changes each week, reinforcing or expanding them gradually. By the end of the eight weeks, you'll be safeguarding your heart and health in a dozen smart ways. And you'll have mastered a repertoire of blood-pressure-lowering techniques that can last you a lifetime.

A note before you begin: Hypertension is serious business. It increases your risk of stroke, heart disease, and kidney disease. So a prudent blood-pressure program should start in your doctor's office, where the two of you can discuss your current diet, exercise level, physical condition, and medical history. Take this program along on your next office visit and go over it with your physician. Get his or her okay before making any changes. If you need to lose a few pounds, decide together on a realistic weight goal. Above all, take your medication faithfully until your doctor tells you to stop or cut back, and have your blood pressure monitored frequently.

Week 1

Start taking 15-minute walks three times a week.   If you walk at a comfortable pace, you'll cover about ¾ mile each time. Exercise is step one in this program because it goes hand-in-hand with weight control—and, as hypertension experts point out, losing excess poundage is the surest nondrug technique for lowering blood pressure.

Drink less alcohol.   Two alcoholic drinks a day, tops. (That's 24 ounces of beer, 8 ounces of wine, or 2 ounces of liquor.) More than that and you risk boosting your blood pressure. In fact, moderation in alcohol intake runs a close second to weight loss in sheer pressure-lowering power, experts say. Heavy drinkers who cut back or quit customarily enjoy a blood pressure drop of several points. Plus, if you're trying to lose weight, the empty calories from alcohol don't help your efforts. So limit yourself or boycott booze entirely.

Tip: If you usually have wine with dinner, make a switch in

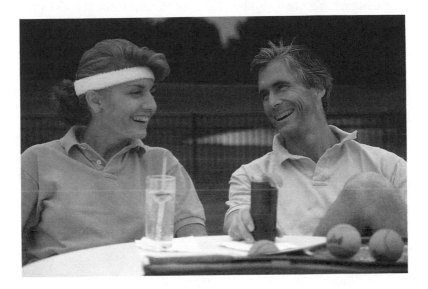

Do you indulge in more than two mixed drinks, two beers, or two glasses of wine a day? If so, you could be boosting your blood pressure. Stick with a two-drink limit. Better yet, skip the spirits. Try an ice-cold, low-sodium seltzer water or a glass of herbal tea...Mmmm, refreshing!

substance—not ambiance. Pour chilled mineral water or salt-free seltzer into wine glasses and add a twist of orange or lemon. Stow the bottle in an ice bucket!

Drink milk every day.   Or eat lots of broccoli. Or low-fat, low-sodium Swiss cheese. Or any combination of these and other foods that'll give you your daily ration of calcium (the Recommended Dietary Allowance, or RDA, is 800 milligrams per day). Research suggests that calcium not only works to keep bones stronger but may also help lower blood pressure in some people.

Tip: If consuming dairy products makes you feel bloated or gassy, you may be lactose intolerant. Try adding enzyme products like Lactaid and Lactase (brand name products available in health-food stores) to milk before drinking. They break down the lactose (milk sugar). You can also buy lactose-reduced milk at some grocery stores.

Bonus Recipe: High-Calcium Stir-Fry

2	large stalks broccoli	2	teaspoons vegetable oil
1	pound tofu*		
	minced garlic and peeled, minced gingerroot, to taste	1	tablespoon low-sodium soy sauce
		2	cups cooked brown rice

In a wok or skillet, stir-fry broccoli, tofu, and seasonings in the vegetable oil. Season with soy sauce and serve hot over brown rice.

Makes 4 servings. (319 calories, 485 milligrams of potassium, 215 milligrams of calcium, and 180 milligrams of sodium per serving)

*Tofu made with calcium sulfate has three times more calcium than nigari-prepared tofu.

Week 2

Increase your walking time to 30 minutes per workout. You should cover about 1½ miles. If this pace is a strain, ease off until you get used to it.

Start eating fish three times a week. Fresh or frozen, baked, broiled, or poached (but never fried), fish is a great catch. Its saturated fat content is usually low, and some fish (like salmon, mackerel, and tuna) score high in omega-3 fatty acids, which seem to have a beneficial effect on risk factors for heart disease. And flounder, cod, haddock, and fresh salmon are good sources of potassium, which has been linked to lower blood pressure and can be depleted by using diuretics.

Limit yourself to one serving of either cured meat or canned soup per week.   Cured meats include bacon, sausage, hot dogs, and luncheon meats—all high-sodium and high-fat items. Canned soups (unless they're labeled otherwise) also pack a lot of sodium. The problem with consuming too much sodium, of course, is that it can raise blood pressure in sodium-sensitive people. Sodium consumption can actually work against many blood-pressure-lowering drugs.

"On the other hand," says Charles P. Tifft, M.D., associate professor of medicine at Boston University's Cardiovascular Institute, "restricting sodium to about 2,000 milligrams per day—the amount found in 1 teaspoon of table salt (sodium chloride)—can lower blood pressure in one hypertensive out of three."

But say your blood pressure never does respond to sodium reduction. Should you feel free to salt up a storm? Sorry—experts think everybody should keep a lid on salt consumption.

Switch to low-fat dairy products.   If you're drinking whole milk, go to 2 percent. If you're drinking 2 percent, try 1 percent. If you're a cheese lover, start enjoying only the low-fat (and low-sodium) varieties. Doing all this can make a big dent in your fat intake. And that can reduce your risk of heart disease and help you keep excess pounds off. After all, fat is loaded with calories—more calories per ounce than either protein or carbohydrates.

Week 3

Increase your walking frequency to five days a week.   The more you exercise, the faster your metabolism works. The faster your metabolism, the more calories your body uses each day, which makes weight loss a whole lot easier.

Stop adding salt when you cook.   Don't add it even

when you're boiling water for pasta. After a while, your taste buds may not even notice the difference.

Turn your thoughts to fruit!   You don't have to give up dessert. Just don't equate dessert with high-sugar, high-fat goodies. Bananas, oranges, cantaloupes, and honeydews are all potassium-rich, calorie-lean, and plenty sweet. Eating out? Ask for a bowl of in-season fruits or fresh fruit sorbet.

Bonus Recipe:
Cool and Fruity Dessert

1 peach, sliced	1 tablespoon lime
1 cup cantaloupe	juice
cubes	½ cup low-fat yogurt
½ cup blueberries	mint leaves, for
1 tablespoon honey,	garnish
warmed	

In a medium bowl, mix peaches, cantaloupe, and blueberries. In a separate container, blend honey, lime juice, and yogurt. Serve fruit mixture in individual dishes and top with yogurt sauce. Garnish with mint leaves.

Makes 2 servings. (138 calories, 512 milligrams of potassium, 118 milligrams of calcium, and 50 milligrams of sodium per serving)

Week 4

Switch to even leaner milk.   If you're drinking 2 percent, try 1 percent. If you're on 1 percent, drink skim. Surprise: One cup of skim milk contains 406 milligrams of potassium (even more than fattier milks), 301 milligrams of calcium, and 127 milligrams of sodium.

Stop salting your food at mealtime.   Instead, fill your saltshaker with your favorite herbs or a no-sodium seasoning and shake away.

Discover the potato!   At least three times a week, have a baked spud or make a potato-based dish. Potatoes are fat-free and loaded with potassium.

Bonus Recipe: Tomato-Potato Salad

1 pound new potatoes, halved	¼ cup minced fresh basil
1 pound tomatoes, cut into chunks	2 teaspoons olive oil

In a large saucepan, steam potatoes until tender, about 8 to 10 minutes. Place in a large bowl and immediately toss with tomatoes, basil, and olive oil. Serve at once, while still warm.

Makes 4 servings. (123 calories, 736 milligrams of potassium, and 18 milligrams of sodium per serving)

Week 5

Pick up the pace.   Aim to cover 2 miles in a half hour if you can do so without strain. You should feel energized by your walks—aches or excessive tiredness are signals to ease up a bit.

Take 10 minutes and relax.   Every day. And we don't mean lie down and worry about tomorrow's workload. But try some serious relaxing by using definite techniques, such as progressive muscle relaxation, meditation, and biofeedback. Research suggests that in some people, these may have a modest, long-term lowering effect on blood pressure.

Week 6

Move beyond walking.   Now's the time to start spicing up your workouts with a little variety—your hedge against exercise boredom and burnout. One or two days a week, skip your walk and swim a few laps at your local pool instead. Or bike around the block. Or whatever. Put in about 15 minutes on each new exercise session and slowly work up to 30 minutes if you can. Don't push and don't overload. You should still be active five days a week.

Be aware, though, that some doctors do not recommend weight machines and weight lifting for people with elevated blood pressure—the effort they require may raise rather than lower blood pressure.

Get into low-sodium snacking.   Ban salty snack foods, such as potato chips, pretzels, and nachos, from your diet. Instead, nosh on unsalted air-popped popcorn, unsalted pretzels, rice cakes, melba toast, or carrots. (Caution: Low-sodium potato and corn chips are high in fat.)

Say yes to yogurt!   And say it three times a week. Plain and simple, yogurt boosts your calcium intake—one low-fat cup dishes out 414 milligrams (that's over half the RDA); spoon up 8 ounces of nonfat and you get 452! Plenty of potassium, too.

Yogurt subs beautifully for fatty no-no's like cream, sour cream, and oil. Browse through low-fat cookbooks for yogurt-based salad dressings, soups, dips, and drinks.

Week 7

Cut out cured meats entirely.   Instead, go for lean cuts of beef, pork, and lamb, along with turkey and chicken. They usually contain less fat and sodium.

Fill up on veggies, three to four servings a day.   Buy them fresh or frozen or look for the reduced-sodium canned variety. Steam or bake or microwave or stir-fry—easy on the oil! Once a week, take a bean to lunch. You probably know that beans are a high-fiber, high-protein food. But did you know that they're also high in potassium?

Bonus Recipe:
Honey-Berry Frozen Yogurt Pops

1   pint fresh   1   teaspoon vanilla
     strawberries   extract
⅓   cup honey   2   cups low-fat yogurt

Place berries in blender or food processor and blend until smooth. Add honey (use less if berries are very sweet), vanilla extract, and yogurt. Blend again.

Pour mixture into ice-pop molds or ice-cube trays, cover with plastic or foil, and freeze for 1 hour; then place wooden sticks in molds. Freeze until solid.

Makes about 1 quart, or 8 ½-cup molds. (92 calories, 202 milligrams of potassium, 110 milligrams of calcium, and 41 milligrams of sodium per serving)

Did you know that some canned beans can have less potassium and 100 over times more sodium than the beans you buy dried and cook yourself? Enough said.

Week 8

Extend your walks to 45 minutes a day.   Cover 2 to 3 miles each time. Continue to substitute other kinds of workouts once in a while. Keep on movin'!

Weigh yourself.   By exercising and following our low-fat, low-salt suggestions, you've probably dropped a few pounds by now—without counting a single calorie. Although a 10-pound loss may produce a drop in blood pressure, it usually takes 20 pounds to make a noticeable difference. Of course, you're best off at your goal weight.

Bonus Recipe:
Three-Bean Salad

1	cup white marrow beans	¼	teaspoon dried oregano
1	cup red kidney beans	½	teaspoon black pepper
1	cup fresh green beans, cut into 1-inch pieces	1	large onion, sliced and separated into rings
1½	tablespoons olive oil	2	stalks celery, sliced thin
3	tablespoons red wine vinegar	2	tablespoons minced parsley
2	cloves garlic, minced		

In a large saucepan, cook the marrow beans and kidney beans, then drain. Place in a large bowl and set aside.

In a medium saucepan, steam green beans for 5 minutes. Add to bowl and set aside.

In a small bowl, mix olive oil, vinegar, garlic, oregano, and pepper. Pour mixture over beans and chill overnight. Before serving, add onion, celery, and parsley. Toss and serve on romaine or other lettuce leaves.

Makes 6 servings. (131 calories, 463 milligrams of potassium, 46 milligrams of magnesium, 67 milligrams of calcium, and 18 milligrams of sodium per serving)

If you have much further to go, talk to your doctor about a long-range weight-loss plan. You may decide to join a support group; self-help organizations can put you on the road to permanent weight loss.

Week 9 and Beyond

Once you have completed the eight-week program outlined in this chapter, there are still some things you should do to maintain your new, healthy lifestyle.

Every Day

- Take your blood pressure medication if it's been prescribed for you.
- Make food choices in line with reaching or maintaining your weight goal.
- Drink less alcohol or none at all. If you do indulge, limit yourself to two drinks.
- Drink milk or eat calcium-rich foods to get your RDA of calcium.
- Stick to low-fat or nonfat dairy products.
- Limit your intake of sodium to 2,000 milligrams (1 teaspoon).
- Eat plenty of fresh fruits and three to four servings of vegetables, including leafy greens and broccoli.
- Take a 10-minute relaxation break.

Five Times a Week (at least)

- Exercise.

Three Times a Week (at least)

- Eat fish.
- Enjoy low-fat, nutritious foods, such as potatoes, yogurt, and whole grains such as brown rice and whole wheat pasta.

Once a Week (at least)

- Eat some beans.

Occasionally

- Weigh yourself.
- Order a sinful dessert.

Evaluate Your Overall Progress

Now how's your blood pressure? Has your doctor reduced your medication? Are you sucessfully limiting alcohol and sodium? You may need more time to make more changes. Don't give up.

When you get in the habit of defusing stress, eating less fat and salt, and exercising each day, at the end of a month or so you may notice the mercury in the blood pressure gauge holding steady at 140 over 90 or lower.

But a lowered blood pressure reading is not a signal to return to your old ways. Once you get your blood pressure low, you have to keep it low by staying on your anti-hypertension program.

You may find it easier to stick with your program if you enlist the support of your entire family. Have them help you find tasty new foods that are less fatty and less salty. Don't keep food in the house that one person can eat but another cannot. Do exercises that other family members can enjoy with you, like walking and bicycling. How about establishing a "walking hour" in place of a cocktail hour? Learn to hear each other out when discussing volatile subjects.

Continue to consult with your doctor as you work toward lower blood pressure—and better health.